Immunology and AIDS Word Book

Helen E. Littrell, CMT

Springhouse
Word Book Series

Springhouse Corporation
Springhouse, Pennsylvania

© Copyright 1992 by
Springhouse Corporation
1111 Bethlehem Pike
Springhouse, Pennsylvania 19477

All rights reserved. No part of this book may be reproduced, stored in a retrieval system or transmitted in any form or by any means, electronic, mechanical, photocopying, recording or otherwise, without written permission from the publisher, except for brief quotations embodied in critical articles and reviews.

Printed in the United States of America

Library of Congress Catalog Card Number: 91-5088

ISBN: 0-87434-475-1

SWB 15-010192

Dedication

To all of those who left us too soon: You dared to follow your dreams and taught us to follow ours.

How to use this book

All entries in this book are listed alphabetically. When a term may be modified in some way with a variety of other terms, the sub-entries are indented and punctuated as follows:
    Abbe-Zeiss (main entry
        counting chamber, A. (main entry comes before sub-entry)
    blood (main entry)
        splanchnic b. (main entry comes after sub-entry)

We've also provided extensive cross-referencing to help you locate certain terms more easily. You'll find this especially valuable when abbreviations may be used interchangeably with the full entry: for example, HIV (human immunodeficiency virus) - also listed as human immunodeficiency virus (HIV).

As an extra value, plural forms of words which change due to Latin origin are shown following the root word: for example, bacillus (pl. bacilli). Bacilli (pl. of bacillus) is also listed alphabetically.

Also included in this book are many coined words and phrases, as well as medical slang, street talk, and the names of controversial drugs and protocols. Because some of these terms are unconventional, you probably will not find them presented in other reference books. This is why we have made many of them part of this book; medical professionals must have a comprehensive reference source for the unique terms that are becoming more and more a part of their daily lives. The fact that they are controversial or unconventional does not mean that they do not exist.

Acknowledgments

Many people deserve thanks for the assistance they provided during the writing of this book — so many that I cannot name all of you. I am grateful to each one for standing by me during some difficult times.

I'm also thankful that Springhouse Corporation has given me the opportunity to write for them. It is indeed a privilege to work with such truly professional people as Jean Robinson and Wendy Clarke.

Additionally, the person who inspired me to write this book deserves the most special thanks of all. He is Brien Ecker, a Stockton, CA physician, whose selfless dedication providing compassionate, skillful medical care to AIDS patients exemplifies the practice of medicine in its finest form. Because Dr. Ecker really cares about the unfortunate victims of this dread disease, his patients receive not only the best of medical care, but — most important of all — dignity and respect.

Thanks also to Project Inform, the San Francisco AIDS Foundation, and many other AIDS information organizations all over the U.S. for enthusiastically providing me with the latest data on experimemtal protocols and regimens, as well as new drugs and food supplements being used in both clinical trials and underground settings. Without the help of these hard-working and cooperative groups, I would have been unable to secure the information needed for this reference.

Most of all, I thank those of you who use this book, because you seek to become more informed about a subject that may eventually touch all of our lives.

Helen E. Littrell, CMT

A

A- (African variant)
A hemoglobin
A68
AA (arachidonic acid)
AAAF (albumin autoagglutinating factor)
Abbe-McIndoe-Williams procedure
Abbe-Zeiss
    cell, A.
    counting cell hemocytometer, A.
    counting chamber, A.
Abbokinase
ABC (antigen-binding capacity)
Abelson
    murine leukemia virus, A.
abetalipoproteinemia
ABGs (arterial blood gases)
ABLC (amphotericin B lipid complex)
ABMA (antibasement membrane antibody)
ABMT (autologous bone marrow transplantation)
ABO (blood group)
    antibodies, A.
    antigens, A.
    compatibility, A.
    erythroblastosis, A.
    incompatibility, A.
    -Rh typing, A.
    typing, A.
ABP (arterial blood pressure)
ABPP
absolute
    basophil count, a.
    eosinophil count, a.
    leukocytosis, a.
    lymphocyte count, a.
    neutrophil count, a.
    reticulocyte count, a.
absorption agglutinin
abstinence
abstinent
ABV (Adriamycin, bleomycin, vinblastine)
ABVD (Adriamycin, bleomycin, vinblastine, dacarbazine)
ACA (anticentromere antibody)
acanthocytes
accelerated
    fractionation, a.
    myeloproliferative phase, a.
accelerator
    factor, a.
    globulin (AcG), a.
accelerin
accessory cell
Accu-Chek II
ACD (acid-citrate-dextrose)
AC/DC (slang for bisexuality)
acetonemia
acetyl glyceryl ether phosphoryl choline (AGEPC)
acetylcholine receptor antibody (AChR-ab)
acetylcholinesterase
AcG (acclerator globulin)
AChRab (acetylcholine receptor antibody)
achrestic anemia
achroacytosis
achromatocyte
achromic erythrocyte
achromocyte
achylanemia
achylic anemia
acid
    agglutination, a.
    -fast bacilli, a. (AFB)
    hematin method, a.
    hemolysis test, a.
    labile alpha interferon, a.
    -lability test, a.
    phosphatase, a. (AP)
    phosphatase RIA, a.
    -Schiff stain, a.
    serum hemolysis, a.
acidemia

acidified serum test
acidocytopenia
acidocytosis
acidophilic erythroblast
acidophilus
acidosis
acidotic
Acinetobacter lwoffi
aclacinomycin
acnemia
acquired
    agammaglobulinemia, a.
    hemolytic anemia, a. (AHA)
    immune deficiency syndrome, a. (AIDS)
    immune hemolytic disease, a. (AIHD)
    immunity, a.
    sideroacrestic anemia, a.
acrocyanosis
acroparesthesia
acrosclerosis
ACS (antireticular cytotoxic serum)
ACT (activated coagulation time)
ACTG (AIDS Clinical Trials Group)
ACTH (adrenocorticotropic hormone)
Actimmune
actinomycin
Activase
activated
    coagulation time, a. (ACT)
    partial thromboplastin time, a. (APTT)
    T-cells, a.
activation factor
active
    immunity, a.
    serum, a.
ACTP (adrenocorticotropic polypeptide)
acupressure
acupuncture
acute
    fulminating toxoplasmosis, a.
    granulocytic leukemia, a. (AGL)
    hemorrhagic leukoencephalitis, a. (AHLE)
    lymphoblastic leukemia, a. (ALL)
    lymphocytic leukemia, a. (ALL)

acute *(continued)*
    monoblastic leukemia, a. (AMOL)
    monocytic leukemia, a. (AML)
    myeloblastic leukemia, a. (AML)
    myelocytic leukemia, a. (AML)
    myelomonoblastic leukemia, a. (AMMOL)
    myelomonocytic leukemia, a. (AMML)
    nonlymphocytic leukemia, a. (ANLL)
    promyelocytic leukemia, a. (APL)
    transforming retrovirus, a.
    tubular necrosis, a.
    undifferentiated leukemia, a. (AUL)
    viral hepatitis, a. (AVH)
ACV (acyclovir)
acycloguanosine
acyclovir (ACV)
ADA (adenosine deaminase)
Adagen
adaptogen
ADC (AIDS dementia complex)
ADCC (antibody-dependent cell-mediated cytotoxicity)
Addis count
addisonian anemia
addisonism
Addison's anemia
Addison-Biermer anemia
adenine arabinoside (Ara-A)
adeno-associated virus
adenosine
    deaminase, a. (ADA)
    kinase, a.
    monophosphate, a. (AMP)
    phosphorylase, a.
    triphosphatase, a.
    triphosphate, a. (ADT or ATP)
    triphosphate pyrophosphohydrolase, a.
adenosinediphosphate deaminase
adenosinetriphosphatase (ATPase)
adenoviral
adenovirus
adherent cell
adhesive platelets
adiemorrhysis

adjuvant
adjuvanticity
AdOAP
adoptive immunity
adrenal
    feminizing syndrome, a.
    gland, a.
    insufficiency, a.
    virilism, a.
    virilizing syndrome, a.
adrenaline
adrenalinemia
adrenalitis
adrenocorticotropic
    hormone, a. (ACTH)
    polypeptide, a. (ACTP)
Adriamycin
ADS (antibody deficiency syndrome)
Adson's maneuver
adsorb
adsorption
ADT (adenosine triphosphate)
adult
    hemoglobin, a.
    T-cell leukemia-lymphoma, a. (ATLL)
ADV (Aleutian disease virus)
adventitial cell
AEF (allogeneic effect factor)
aerobe
    obligate a.
aerobic
    diphtheroids, a.
AeroChamber
Aeropent
Aeroseb-Dex
aerosol
aerosolization
aerosolized pentamidine (AP)
Aerosporin
AF (antibody-forming)
AFB (acid-fast bacilli)
AFC (antibody-forming cells)
afferentia
affinity
    chromatography, a.
    labeling, a.

afflux
afibrinogenemia
afibrogenemia
AFP (alpha-fetoprotein)
African
    Burkitt lymphoma, A.
    green monkey, A.
    Kaposi's sarcoma, A.
    lymphoma, A.
    (A-) variant, A.
Ag (antigen)
agammaglobulinemia (AGG)
    acquired a.
    Bruton's a.
    common variable a.
    congenital a.
    lymphopenic a.
    Swiss-type a.
    X-linked a.
    X-linked infantile a.
agar
    gel electrophoresis, a.
Agar-IF (immunofixation in agar)
agarose
agent
AGEPC (acetyl glyceryl ether phosphoryl choline)
AGG (agammaglobulinemia)
agglutin
agglutinant
agglutination
    acid a.
    bacteriogenic a.
    cold a.
    cross-a.
    group a.
    H a.
    intravascular a.
    macroscopic a.
    microscopic a.
    O a.
    passive a.
    platelet a.
    salt a.
    spontaneous a.
    Vi a.

agglutinator
agglutinin
    absorption a.
    anti-Rh a.
    chief a.
    cold a.
    complete a.
    cross a.
    flagellar a.
    group a.
    H a.
    immune a.
    incomplete a.
    leukocyte a.
    major a.
    MG a.
    minor a.
    O a.
    partial a.
    platelet a.
    saline a.
    somatic a.
    T a.
    warm a.
agglutinin absorption
agglutinin adsorption
agglutinogen
    A and B a.
    M and N a.
    Rh a.
agglutinogenic
agglutinophilic
agglutometer
aggregate
aggregated human IgG (AHuG)
aggregation
aggregometer
aggregometry
aggressin
AGL (acute granulocytic leukemia)
aglycemia
agnocobalamin
agnogenic myeloid metaplasia (AMM)
agonal
    leukocytosis, a.
agonist

agranulocytic
agranulocytosis
A/G ratio (albumin/globulin ratio)
agretope
AGT (antiglobulin test)
AHA (acquired OR autoimmune hemolytic anemia)
ahaptoglobinemia
AHF (antihemophilic factor)
AHG (antihemophilic globulin OR antihuman globulin)
AHLE (acute hemorrhagic leukoencephalitis)
AHLS (antihuman lymphocyte serum)
AHuG (aggregated human IgG)
AIDS (acquired immune deficiency syndrome)
    arthritis, A.
    Clinical Trials Group, A. (ACTG)
    dementia complex, A. (ADC)
    enteropathy, A.
    psychosis, A.
    -related complex, A. (ARC)
    -related disease, A. (ARD)
    -related syndrome, A (ARS)
    -related virus, A. (ARV)
AIHA (autoimmune hemolytic anemia)
AIHD (acquired immune hemolytic disease)
AIL (angioimmunoblastic lymphadenopathy)
AILD (angioimmunoblastic lymphadenopathy with dysproteinemia)
AIO (amyloid of immunoglobulin origin)
AIP (automated immunoprecipitation)
airborne
AITP (autoimmune thrombocytopenic purpura)
akaryocyte
akaryote
akembe
alanine aminotransferase (ALT)
albukalin
albumin
    autoagglutinating factor, a. (AAAF)
    -bound dye, a.

albumin *(continued)*
    globulin ratio, a. (A/G ratio)
    quotient, a.
Albuminar
albuminemia
albumose plasma
Albumotope
alcaptonuria-ochronosis
Alcian blue
Alcobon
alcoholemia
alcoholism
aldo-keto reductase
Aldrich syndrome
aleukemia
aleukemic
    leukemia, a.
aleukia
    hemorrhagica, a.
aleukocythemic leukemia
aleukocytic
aleukocytosis
Aleutian disease virus (ADV)
Alexan
alexin
alfacalcidol
Alferon
    -N, A.
    -N-Injection, A.
ALG (antilymphocyte globulin)
alimentary toxemia
aliphatic series
alkalating
alkalemia
alkali reserve
alkalimetry
alkaline phosphatase (ALP)
alkaloid
alkalosis
alkalotic
ALL (acute lymphoblastic OR lympho-
    cytic leukemia)
allele
allelic
    exclusion, a.
    gene, a.

allelomorph
Allen's treatment
allergen
allergenic
allergic
    reaction, a.
allergization
allergy
    atopic a.
    bacterial a.
    bronchial a.
    cold a.
    contact a.
    delayed a.
    drug a.
    food a.
    gastrointestinal a.
    hereditary a.
    immediate a.
    latent a.
    physical a.
    pollen a.
    polyvalent a.
    spontaneous a.
    total a.
allesthesia
alloagglutinin
alloalbuminemia
alloantibody
alloantigen
alloantin-D antibody
allogeneic
    effect factor, a. (AEF)
allogenic
    bone marrow transplant, a.
allograft
allogroup
alloimmune
alloimmunization
allopurinol
allosensitization
allosterism
allotoxin
allotype
    Am a.
    Gm a.

allotype *(continued)*
   Inv a.
   Km a.
   Oz a.
allotypic
   determinant, a.
   variant, a.
allotypy
alloxan-Schiff reaction
alloxantin
alloxuremia
alopecia
ALP (alkaline phosphatase OR antilymphocyte plasma)
alpha
   cell, a.
   chain, a.
   chain disease, a.
   chain thalassemia, a.
   -difluoromethylornithine, a.
   -fetoglobin, a.
   -fetoprotein, a. (AFP)
   globulin, a.
   granules, a.
   HCD, a.
   heavy chain disease, a.
   -helix, a.
   hemoglobin, a.
   interferon, a.
   macroglobulin, a.
   -2-macroglobulin, a.
   -methyldopa, a.
   -methylparatyrosine, a.
   -1-thymosin, a.
alphavirus
ALS (antilymphocyte serum)
AL-721
ALT (alanine aminotransferase)
alteplase
Altrigen
ALT-RCC (autolymphocyte-based treatment for renal cell carcinoma)
alum
   hematoxylin, a.
   -precipitated antigen, a.
alymphocytosis

ALZ-50
AM allotype
amanita toxin
amantadine hydrochloride
Amapari virus
Amato bodies
ambiguous genitalia
Ambisome
amboceptor unit
AME (amphotericin methyl ester)
amebiasis
   hemagglutination titer, a.
American Rolland
Ames assay
AMF (autocrine motility factor)
AmFAR (The American Foundation for AIDS Research)
AMG (antimacrophage globulin)
Amicar
amikacin
amine
amino acid
aminoacidemia
aminoacidopathy
aminobutyrate aminotransferase
aminocaproic acid
aminogram
aminotransferase
AML (acute monocytic OR myelocytic OR monoblastic leukemia)
AMLS (antimouse lymphocyte serum)
AMM (agnogenic myeloid metaplasia)
AMML (acute myelomonocytic leukemia)
AMMOL (acute myelomonoblastic leukemia)
ammonemia
AMOL (acute monoblastic leukemia)
AMP (adenosine monophosphate)
amphetamine
amphileukemic
amphoteric electrolyte
amphotericin B
   B lipid complex, a. (ABLC)
amphotericin methyl ester (AME)
amplifier T-lymphocyte
Ampligen

AMS (antimacrophage serum)
amsacrine
Amsidyl
amygdalin
amyl nitrite (popper)
amylase
amylemia
amyloid
    immunoglobulin origin, a. of (AIO)
    L-chain, a.
amyloidogenic protein
amyloidosis
ANA (antinuclear antibodies)
anabolic steroid
anachoretic effect
anaerobe
anaerobic
    diphtheroids, a.
anal
    canal, a.
    copulation, a.
    crypt, a.
    eroticism, a.
    fisting, a.
    intercourse, a.
    phase, a.
    rimming, a.
    sadism, a.
    sex, a.
    stage, a.
anallergenic serum
analogue
anamnestic response
anaphylactic
    shock, a.
anaphylactoid
    crisis, a.
    purpura, a.
    reaction, a.
anaphylatoxin
anaphylaxis
anaplasmosis vaccine
anatoxic
anatoxin
    -Ramon, a.
Ancobon

Ancotil
androgen
anemia
    achrestic a.
    achylic a.
    acquired sideroachrestic a.
    acute a.
    Addison's a.
    Addison-Biermer a.
    addisonian a.
    anhematopoietic a.
    aplastic a.
    aregenerative a.
    autoimmune hemolytic a. (AIHA)
    Bagdad Spring a.
    Bartonella a.
    Biermer's a.
    Biermer-Ehrlich a.
    Blackfan-Diamond a.
    cameloid a.
    cancer-associated a.
    chlorotic a.
    Chvostek's a.
    congenital a. of newborn
    congenital dyserythropoietic a.
    congenital hypoplastic a.
    congenital nonspherocytic
        hemolytic a.
    Cooley's a.
    cow's milk a.
    crescent cell a.
    cytogenic a.
    deficiency a.
    dilution a.
    dimorphic a.
    drepanocytic a.
    Dresbach's a.
    drug-induced immune hemolytic a.
    dyserythropoietic a.
    Edelmann's a.
    elliptocytary a.
    elliptocytotic a.
    erythroblastic a. of childhood
    erythronormoblastic a.
    essential a.
    Estren-Damashek a.

anemia *(continued)*
    familial erythroblastic a.
    familial megaloblastic a.
    Fanconi's a.
    folic acid deficiency a.
    globe cell a.
    glucose-6-phosphate dehydrogenase deficiency a.
    goat's milk a.
    ground itch a.
    Heinz body hemolytic a.
    hemolytic a.
    hemorrhagic a.
    hereditary nonspherocytic hemolytic a.
    Herrick's a.
    hookworm a.
    hypersplenic a.
    hypochromic a.
    hypochromic microcytic a.
    hypoferric a.
    hypoplastic a.
    iatrogenic a.
    icterohemolytic a.
    idiopathic a.
    idiopathic hypochromic a.
    immune hemolytic a.
    infectious hemolytic a.
    intertropical a.
    iron deficiency a.
    Jaksch's a.
    Lederer's a.
    leukoerythroblastic a.
    macrocytic a.
    Mediterranean a.
    megaloblastic a.
    megalocytic a.
    microangiopathic a.
    microangiopathic hemolytic a.
    microcytic a.
    microdrepanocytic a.
    milk a.
    miner's a.
    mountain a.
    myelopathic a.
    myelophthisic a.
    neonatorum, a.

anemia *(continued)*
    normochromic a.
    normocytic a.
    nosocomial a.
    nutritional a.
    nutritional macrocytic a.
    osteosclerotic a.
    pernicious a.
    phenylhydrazine a.
    physiologic a.
    polar a.
    posthemorrhagic a.
    posthemorrhagic a. of newborn
    primaquine-sensitive a.
    primary a.
    protein deficiency a.
    pseudoleukemica infantum, a.
    pure red cell a.
    pyridoxine-responsive a.
    refractoria sideroblastica, a.
    refractory a.
    refractory sideroblastic a.
    Runeberg's a.
    scorbutic a.
    secondary a.
    septic a.
    sickle cell a.
    siderachrestic a.
    sideroblastic a.
    sideropenic a.
    simple achlorhydric a.
    slaty a.
    spherocytic a.
    splenic a.
    spur-cell a.
    thrombopenic a.
    toxic hemolytic a.
    traumatic cardiac hemolytic a.
    tropic a.
    tropical macrocytic a.
    vitamin deficiency a.
    Von Jaksch's a.
anemic
    hypoxia, a.
    necrosis, a.
anergic

anergy
   panel, a.
anerythroplasia
ANF (antinuclear factor)
angel dust (PCP)
angioaccess
angioataxia
angiodermatitis
angioedema
angiogenesis
angiohemophilia
angioimmunoblastic lymphadenopathy (AIL)
   dysproteinemia, a. with (AILD)
angiopressure
angiosthenia
angiostomy
angiotelectasis
angiotensin
   -I converting enzyme, a.
angiotensinase
angiotensinogen
anhematopoietic anemia
anikacin sulfate
anilingus
anilinism
animal
   toxin, a.
   virus, a.
anion gap
anisocytosis
anisohypercytosis
anisohypocytosis
anisokaryosis
anisoleukocytosis
anisonormocytosis
anisoylated plasminogen streptokinase activator complex (APSAC)
anistreplase (Eminase)
ANLL (acute nonlymphocytic leukemia)
Ann Arbor classification
annular
   phased array EMW hyperthermia, a.
   thrombus, a.
anonymous mycobacterium
anorectal

anorectal *(continued)*
   herpes, a.
   syphilis, a.
anorectum
anoxemia
anoxia
ANS (antineutrophilic serum)
ansamycin (LM427)
Ansbacher unit
Antabuse
antagonist
antherpetic
anthocyanin
anthocyaninemia
anthracenediones
anthracycline
anthrax
   spore vaccine, a.
   toxin, a.
Anthron heparinized catheter
antiacetylcholine receptor (anti-AChR) antibodies
anti-AChr (antiacetylcholine receptor) antibodies
antiagglutinin
antianaphylaxis
antianemia principle
antianemic factor
antiantibody
antiantidote
anti-anti-Factor VIII
antiantitoxin
antiautolysin
antibacterial
   immunity, a.
antibasement membrane antibody, a. (ABMA)
antibody
   ABO a.
   acetylcholine receptor a.
   alloantin-D a.
   anaphylactic a.
   antiacetylcholine receptor, a. (anti-AChrR)
   anticentromere a.
   anticytoplasmic a.

antibody *(continued)*
    anti-D a.
    anti-DNA a.
    antifibrin a.
    antiglomerular basement membrane,
        a. (anti-GEM)
    anti-idiotype a.
    anti-Leu 3a a.
    antimicrosomal a.
    antimitochondrial a.
    antinuclear a.
    antipeptide a.
    antireceptor a.
    anti-Ro a.
    anti-Sm a.
    anti-T-cell a.
    antithyroglobulin a.
    antithyroid a.
    auto-anti-idiotypic a.
    autologous a.
    bispecific a.
    blocking a.
    cell-bound a.
    cell-fixed a.
    cell-mediated a.
    cold a.
    cold-reactive a.
    combining-site a.
    complement-fixing a.
    complete a.
    cross-reacting a.
    cryptosporidiosis a.
    cytophilic a.
    cytotoxic a.
    cytotropic a.
    Donath-Landsteiner a.
    duck virus hepatitis yolk a.
    Duffy a.
    enhancing a.
    fluorescent a.
    Forssman a.
    HBcAb a.
    HBeAb a.
    HBsAb a.
    heteroclitic a.
    heterogenetic a.

antibody *(continued)*
    heterophil a.
    heterophile a.
    hemocytotropic a.
    humoral a.
    hybrid a.
    hybridoma a.
    IgM-RF a.
    immune a.
    incomplete a.
    isophil a.
    Kell a.
    Kidd a.
    Lewis a.
    Lutheran a.
    maternal a.
    mitochondrial a.
    monoclonal a.
    natural a.
    neutralizing a.
    nonprecipitation a.
    opsonizing a.
    Ortho-mune a.
    P-K a.
    polyclonal a.
    Prausnitz-Kustner a.
    protective a.
    reaginic a.
    Rh a.
    saline a.
    sensitizing a.
    skin-sensitizing a.
    TSH-displacing a.
    warm a.
    warm-reactive a.
antibody catabolism
antibody-coated bacteria
antibody deficiency syndrome (ADS)
antibody-dependent cell-mediated cyto-
    toxicity (ADCC)
antibody-forming (AF)
antibody-forming cells (AFC)
antibody half-life
antibody molecules
antibody titer
anti-C antibody

anticentromere antibody (ACA)
anticholera serum
anticholesteremic
anticipatory immune suppression
anticoagulant
anticoagulate
anticoagulative
anticodon
anticomplement
anticomplementary
   serum, a.
anticrotalus serum
anticytolysin
anticytoplasmic
anticytotoxin
anti-D antibody
antidiphtheritic serum
anti-E antibody
anti-EA antibody
anti-factor disorder
antifibrin antibody
antifibrinogen
antifibrinolysin
antifibrinolytic
antifol
antifolate
antifolic
antifungal
anti-Fy (Duffy) antibody
anti-GEM (antiglomerular basement
   membrane) antibodies
antigen (Ag)
   acetone-insoluble a.
   allogeneic a.
   alum-precipitated a.
   Am a.
   Au a.
   Australia a.
   bacterial a.
   B-cell differentiation a.
   beef heart a.
   blood-group a.
   Boivin a.
   CA-125 a.
   capsular a.
   carcinoembryonic a. (CEA)

antigen (Ag) *(continued)*
   Chido-Rodgers a.
   cholesterinized a.
   class I a.
   class II a.
   class III a.
   common a.
   common acute lymphoblastic leukemia a. (CALLA)
   common leukocyte a.
   complete a.
   conjugated a.
   cross-reacting a.
   cryptococcal a.
   D a.
   delta a.
   differentiation a.
   Duffy a.
   E a.
   early a.
   endogenous a.
   exogenous a.
   extractable nuclear a. (ENA)
   febrile a.
   flagellar a.
   Forssman a.
   Frei a.
   Gm a.
   H a.
   hepatitis a.
   hepatitis-associated a. (HAA)
   hepatitis B core a.
   hepatitis B e a.
   hepatitis B surface a.
   heterogeneic a.
   heterogenetic a.
   heterologous a.
   heterophil a.
   heterophile a.
   histocompatibility a.
   HLA (human leukocyte OR lymphocyte)
   homologous a.
   H-2 a.
   human leukocyte a. (HLA)
   human lymphocyte a. (HLA)

antigen (Ag) *(continued)*
   human thymus lymphocyte a.
   H-Y a.
   Ia a.
   idiotypic a.
   inhalant a.
   Inv group a.
   isogeneic a.
   isophile a.
   K a.
   Km a.
   Kveim a.
   LD a.
   leukocyte common a.
   Ly a.
   Lyb a.
   lymphocyte-defined (LD) a.
   lymphogranuloma venereum a.
   Lyt a.
   M a.
   Mitsuda a.
   mumps skin test a.
   nuclear a.
   O a.
   oncofetal a.
   organ-specific a.
   Oz a.
   pancreatic oncofetal a. (POA)
   partial a.
   PHA (phytohemagglutinin) a.
   phytohemagglutinin a.
   plasma cell a.
   pollen a.
   Pr a.
   private a.
   proliferating cell nuclear a.
   public a.
   QA a.
   recall a.
   Rh factor a.
   SD a.
   self-a.
   sequestered a.
   serodefined a.
   serologically defined a.
   serum hepatitis a.

antigen (Ag) *(continued)*
   SH a.
   shock a.
   skin-specific histocompatibility a.
   Sm a.
   somatic a.
   species-specific a.
   SS-A a.
   SS-B a.
   surface a.
   synthetic a.
   T a.
   Tac a.
   T-cell a.
   T-cell differentiation a.
   T-dependent a.
   theta a.
   Thy 1 a.
   thymus-dependent a.
   thymus-independent a.
   T-independent a.
   tissue-specific a.
   TL a.
   transplantation a.
   tumor-associated a.
   tumor-specific a.
   tumor-specific transplantation a. (TSTA)
   VDRL a.
   Vi a.
   viral capsid a.
   xenogeneic a.
antigen-antibody reaction
antigen-binding capacity (ABC)
antigen-binding site
antigen-combining site
antigen gain
antigen-presenting site
antigen-reactive cell
antigen-sensitive cell
antigen unit
antigenemia
antigenic
   antibody lattice formation, a.
   binding receptor, a.
   determinant, a.

antigenic *(continued)*
    drift, a.
    modulation, a.
    reversible, a.
    shift, a.
    variation, a.
antigenicity
antigenotherapy
antiglobulin
    consumption test, a.
    test, a. (AGT)
antiglomerular basement membrane (anti-GEM) antibodies
antigrowth factor
anti-G suit
anti-HBc
anti-HBs
antihemagglutinin
antihemolysin
antihemolytic
antihemophilia
    factor, a. (factor VIII)
antihemophilic
    factor, a. (AHF)
    globulin, a. (AHG)
    human plasma, a.
antihemorrhagic
    factor, a.
    vitamin, a.
antihepatic serum
antiheterolysin
antihistamine
antihistone
anti-HIV
    immune serum globulin, a. (HIVIG)
antihormone
antihuman
    globulin, a. (AHG)
    lymphocyte serum, a. (AHLS)
antihypercholesterolemic
antihyperglycemic
antihyperlipoproteinemic
antihypertensive
antihypotensive
anti-Ia serum
anti-icteric

anti-idiotype
anti-immunoglobulin
anti-infective
anti-intercellular
anti-interferon immunoglobulin
anti-K (Kell) antiboy
antiketogenesis
anti-KI (Kidd) antibody
antikinase
anti-La antibody
anti-Leu-2A antibody
anti-Leu-3A antibody
antileukemic
antileukocidin
antileukocytic
antileukoprotease
antilipemic
antilymphocyte
    globulin, a. (ALG)
    plasma, a. (ALP)
    serum, a. (ALS)
antimacrophage
    globulin, a. (AMG)
    serum, a. (AMS)
antimeningococcal
    serum, a.
antimetabolite
antimethemoglobinemic
antimicrobial
antimitochondral
antimoniotungstate
antimonium tungstate (HPA-23)
antimouse lymphocyte serum (AMLS)
antimuscle antibody
antimycobacterial
antineoplastic
antineutrophilic
    cytoplasmic antibody, a.
    serum, a. (ANS)
antinuclear
    antibodies, a. (ANA)
    factor, a. (ANF)
anti-P antibody
antiparietal
anti-pernicious anemia factor
antipertussis serum

antiphagocytic
antiphthisic
antiplaque serum
antiplasmin
antiplastic
antiplatelet
    autoantibodies, a.
    serum, a.
antipneumococcal
    serum, a.
antipneumocystis
antipolycythemic
antiprecipitin
antiprothrombin
antiprotozoal
anti-Pseudomonas human plasma (APHP)
antirabies serum
antireticular cytotoxic serum (ACS)
antiretroviral
anti-Rh agglutinin
anti-RHO-D titer
anti-Ro antibody
antiscarlatinal serum
antiscorbutic factor
antisense
    DNA sequence, a.
    oligodeoxynucleotide, a.
antisera (pl. of antiserum)
antiserum (pl. antisera)
antisheep
    erythrocyte antibody, a.
    red blood cells, a.
antishock suit
anti-Sm (Smith) antibody
antistaphyloccal
    serum, a.
antistaphylolysin
antistreptococcal
    hyaluronidase, a. (ASH)
    serum, a.
antistreptococcic
antistreptococcin
antistreptokinase (ASK)
antistreptolysin (AS)
    O, a. (ASO)
antitetanic serum
antithrombin
    III, a. (ATnativ)
antithromboplastic
antithrombotic
antithymocyte
    globulin, a. (ATG)
    serum, a. (ATS)
antithyroglobulin (ATG)
antitoxic
    immunity, a.
    serum, a.
    unit, a.
antitoxin
antitoxinogen
antitropin
antitrypanosomal
antitubular basement membrane antibodies
antityphoid serum
antivenom
antivenomous serum
antivimenten
antiviral
    immunity, a.
antivirotic
Antrypol
anus
anusitis
AP (acid phosphatase OR aerosolized pentamidine)
apatite-associated large joint lysis
APC (antigen-presenting cell)
    virus, A.
apeu virus
apheresis
APHP (anti-Pseudomonas human plasma)
aphtha (pl. aphthae)
aphthae (pl. of aphtha)
aphthous
    stomatitis, a.
    ulcer, a.
aphthovirus
APL (acute promyelocytic leukemia)
aplasia
aplastic
    anemia, a.

aplastic *(continued)*
   crisis, a.
apolipoprotein
APPG (aqueous procaine penicillin G)
appropriate polycythemia
APSAC (anisoylated plasminogen streptokinase activator complex)
Apt test
APTT (activated partial thromboplastin time)
apurinic acid
Aqua-Mephyton
aqueous vaccine
Ara-A (adenine arabinoside)
Arabitin
Ara-C (cytosine arabinoside)
arachidonate
arachidonic acid (AA)
Aralen
arborizing
arborvirus
arboviral
arbovirus
ARC (AIDS-related complex)
archoptosis
archorrhagia
archorrhea
arctic anemia
ARD (AIDS-related disease)
aregenerative anemia
Arenaviridae
arenavirus
argatroban
Argentinian hemorrhagic fever
arginase
argininemia
argininosuccinicacidemia
argyremia
armed macrophage
Arneth count
Arnold's bodies
ARS (AIDS-related syndrome)
ART (automated reagin test)
artemesia annua
arterial
   blood, a.

arterial *(continued)*
   blood gases, a. (ABGs)
   blood pressure, a. (ABP)
   circulation, a.
   line, a.
arteriovenous (AV)
   fistula, a. (AVF)
arthritis
   atypical mycobacterial a.
   bacterial a.
   candidal a.
   degenerative a.
   enteropathic a.
   erosive a.
   fungal a.
   gonococcal a.
   gouty a.
   gram-negative bacilli a.
   hemochromatotic a.
   infectious a.
   inflammatory a.
   meningococcal a.
   monoarticular a.
   mutilans, a.
   mycobacterial a.
   neuropathic a.
   nongonococcal bacterial a.
   psoriatic a.
   pyogenic a.
   reactive a.
   rheumatoid a.
   rubella a.
   sarcoid a.
   septic a.
   traumatic a.
   tuberculous a.
   viral a.
arthropathy
Arthus reaction
artificial
   blood, a.
   immunity, a.
   kidney, a.
   leech, a.
ARV (AIDS-related virus)
arylsulfatase

AS (antistreptolysin)
Asacol
Aschoff
  bodies, A.
  cells, A.
ascorbemia
ascorbic acid
aseptic meningitis
ASH (antistreptococcal hyaluronidase)
A68
ASK (antistreptokinase)
ASO (antistreptolysin O)
  titer, A.
AS-101 (ammonium trichlorotellurate)
L-asparagine
  -linked oligosaccharide, a.
aspartate
  aminotransferase, a. (AST)
  carbamoyl transferase, a.
  transaminase, a.
aspergilloma
aspergillosis
Aspergillus
assay
  biological a.
  blastogenesis a.
  cell-mediated lympholysis a.
  CH 50 a.
  complement a.
  E rosette a.
  EAC rosette a.
  ELISA a.
  enzyme-linked immunosorbent a. (ELISA)
  four-point a.
  hemagglutination inhibition a.
  hemolytic complement a.
  hemolytic plaque a.
  immune a.
  immune adherence hemagglutination a.
  immunofluorescent a.
  immunoradiometric a.
  Jerne plaque a.
  leukotactic a.
  lymphocyte proliferation a.

assay *(continued)*
  microbiological a.
  microcytotoxicity a.
  microhemagglutination a. - Treponema pallidum (MHA-TP)
  mixed lymphocyte culture a.
  plaque-forming cell a.
  polyethylene glycol precipitation a.
  radioligand a.
  radioreceptor a.
  Raji cell a.
  RAST inhibition a.
  staphylococcal protein A binding a.
  stem cell a.
  total complement a.
  Treponema pallidum hemagglutination a. (TPHA)
  whole complement a.
association constant
AST (aspartate aminotransferase)
asteroid bodies
asthenia
Astrup blood gas values
Asuro
asymptomatic
  seropositive, a.
  shedding, a.
AS-l0l (ammonium trichlorotellurate)
ATG (antithymocyte globulin OR antithyroglobulin)
Athrombin-K
athyroidemia
ATLL (adult T-cell leukemia-lymphoma)
ATLV (adult T-cell leukemia virus)
ATnativ (antithrombin III)
atopic allergy
Atopicide
atopy
ATP (adenosine triphosphate)
  pyrophosphohydrolase, A.
ATPase (adenosinetriphosphatase)
atransferrinemia
ATS (antithymocyte serum)
attenuated
  vaccine, a.
  virus, a.

Attenuvax
Atvogen
atypical
   lymphocyte, a.
   Mycobacteria, a.
   mycobacterial arthritis, a.
Au (Australia)
   Ag, A. (Australia antigen)
   antigen, A.
   antigenemia, A.
Auer bodies
AUL (acute undifferentiated leukemia)
auranofin
aurotherapy
Austin and VanSlyke's method
Australia
   antigen assay, A.
   (Au) antigen, A.
Australian
   Q fever, A.
   X disease virus, A.
Autenrieth and Funk's method
autoadsorption
autoagglutination
autoagglutinin
autoallergic
autoallergy
autoantibody
autoanticomplement
autoantigen
autoantitoxin
autobody
Autoclix
autocrine motility factor (AMF)
autocytolysin
autoerythrocyte sensitization
autoerythrophagocytosis
autofluorescence
autogenic
   graft, a.
autogenous
autograft
autohemagglutination
autohemagglutinin
autohemolysin
autohemolysis
autohemolytic
autohemotherapy
autohemotransfusion
autoimmune
   hemolytic anemia, a. (AHA or AIHA)
   leukopenia, a.
   pancytopenia, a.
   polyendocrine-candidiasis syndrome, a.
   reaction, a.
   response, a.
   thrombocytopenic purpura, a. (AITP)
   thyroiditis, a.
autoimmunity
autoimmunization
autoinfection
autoinfusion
autoinoculable
autoinoculation
autointerference
autoisolysin
Autolet
autoleukoagglutinin
autologous
   blood, a.
   bone marrow transplantation, a. (ABMT)
   clot, a.
   graft, a.
   hematopoietic reconstitution, a.
   transfusion, a.
autolymphocyte
   -based treatment for renal cell carcinoma, a. (ALT-RCC)
autolysin
autolysis
automated
   immunoprecipitation, a. (AIP)
   reagin test, a. (ART)
Autoplex
autoprothrombin
autoradiography
autoreinfusion
autosensitization
autosensitized
autoserotherapy

autoserum
autosomal gene
autotherapy
autothromboagglutinin
autotoxemia
autotoxic
autotoxicosis
autotoxin
autotransfusion
autotuberculin
autovaccination
autovaccine
autovaccinia
autovaccinotherapy
autoxemia
AV (arteriovenous)
    fistula, A.
avarol
avarone
AVF (arteriovenous fistula)
AVH (acute viral hepatitis)
aviadenovirus
avian
    E26 virus, a.
    erythroblastosis virus, a.
    leukemia virus, a.
    leukosis virus, a.
    myeloblastosis virus, a.
    tuberculosis antigen, a.

avian *(continued)*
    virus E, a.
avidin
avipoxvirus
avirulent
Avitene
Avlosulfon (dapsone)
axoplasmic
ayw1, ayw2, ayw4, aywr (hepatitis B surface antigen subdeterminants)
azaribine
azathioprine
6-azauridine
AzdU (azidouridine)
azidodideoxyuridine
azidothymidine (AZT)
azidouridine (AzdU)
Azimexon
aziridinylbenzoquinone (AZQ)
azithromycin
Azlin
azotemia
AZQ (aziridinylbenzoquinone)
AZT (azidothymidine)
aztreonam
azur granules
azurophil granules
azurophilia

Additional entries

B

BA (blocking antibody)
Babesia microti
babesiosis
BAC (blood alcohol concentration)
bacillemia
bacilli (pl. of bacillus)
bacillus (pl. bacilli)
bacteremia
bacteria (pl. of bacterium)
bacterial
   antagonism, b.
   arthritis, b.
   resistance, b.
   toxin, b.
   vaccine, b.
   virus, b.
bactericidal
bactericide
bactericidin
bacterid
bacterin-toxoid
bacterioagglutinin
bacteriogenic
   agglutination, b.
bacteriohemagglutinin
bacteriohemolysin
bacteriolysin
bacteriolysis
bacteriolytic
   serum, b.
bacteriophage
bacteriophagia
bacteriopsonin
bacteriostasis
bacteriostatic
bacteriotoxemia
bacteriotropin
bacterium (pl. bacteria)
BactoAgar
Bactrim
baculovirus
Bafverstedt syndrome
Bagdad Spring anemia

Baker's acid hematein test
BALB/c sarcoma virus
ball thrombus
balloon cells
band
   cells, b.
   form, b.
   neutrophil, b.
bandemia
bands
Banti disease
B1 antibody
B2 antibody
BAP (blood agar plate)
barbiturate
barbiturism
Barcroft's apparatus
bare lymphocyte syndrome
Bareggi's reaction
Bargen's streptococcus
Barlow's disease
barrier
   method, b.
Barron pump
Bart's hemoglobin
Bartonella anemia
bartonellosis
Bartter syndrome
base
   deficit, b.
   excess, b.
   pair, b.
baseline
basic
   calcium phosphate, b. (BCP)
   fibroblast growth factor, b. (bFGF)
Basidiomycetes
basocyte
basocytopenia
basocytosis
basoerythrocyte
basoerythrocytosis
basopenia

basophil
   chemotactic factor, b. (BCF)
basophilia
basophilic
   cell, b.
   erythroblast, b.
   erythrocyte, b.
   leukemia, b.
   leukocyte, b.
   leukocytosis, b.
   series, b.
   stippling, b.
basophilism
Bay region concept
BBB (blood-brain barrier)
BCDF (B-cell differentiation factor)
B-cell
   associated antigen, B.
   differentiation factor, B, (BCDF)
   growth factor, B. (BCGF)
   lymphoma, B.
   mitogen, B.
   restricted antigen, B.
BCF (basophil chemotactic factor)
BCG (bacille Calmette-Guerin)
   vaccine, B.
BCGF (B-cell growth factor)
BCP (basic calcium phosphate)
Bearn-Kunkel-Slater syndrome
bed
   blocking, b.
   blocks, b.
   -bound, b.
bedfast
bee sting kit
beef heart antigen
Behcet's disease
Behring's law
Belganyl
Bence Jones
   albumin, B.
   bodies, B.
   myeloma, B.
   protein, B.
   proteinuria, B.
   reaction, B.

benign
   monoclonal gammopathy, b. (BMG)
   polycythemia, b.
Bennett classification
benoxaprofen
benzidine test
berdache
Berkefeld filter
Bernard-Soulier syndrome
berry cells
Berry-Dedrick phenomenon
Bessey-Lowry units
Bestatin
bestiality
beta
   basophil, b.
   cells, b.
   finger grip, b.
   globulin, b.
   hemolysis, b.
   -hemolytic streptococcus, b.
   interferon, b.
   lipoprotein, b.
   -lysin, b.
   -microglobulin, b.
   -2-microglobulin, b. (B2MG)
   -pleated sheet, b.
   -propiolactone, b.
   thalassemia, b.
   -thromboglobulin, b.
Betaseron
Bethesda unit
BF (blastogenic factor)
bFGF (basic fibroblast growth factor)
BFP (biologic false-positive)
BFU-E (burst-forming unit-erythroid)
bG (blood glucose)
BGG (bovine gamma globulin)
BGSA (blood granulocyte-specific activity)
BHT (butylated hydroxytoluene)
BH/VH (body hematocrit/venous hematocrit ratio)
Bicarbolyte
bicarbonatemia
Bicibon

Biermer's anemia
Biermer-Ehrlich anemia
bile salts
Bili light
bilirubin
bilirubinemia
binding
    constant, b.
    protein, b.
Binelli's styptic
bioassay
    -mouse thyroid stimulation in vivo, b.
bioavailability
biochemical
    marker, b.
    racial index, b.
biofeedback
biogenesis
biogenetic
biologic
    false-positive, b. (BFP)
    markers, b.
biological
    assay, b.
    half-life, b.
    response modifiers, b. (BRMs)
biosmosis
biostimulation
biotin
    -avidin-peroxidase im-
        munoperoxidase, b.
biovar
biovariance
biovariant
biphosphoglycerate phosphatase
Birbeck granule
bird's nest filter
BI-RG-587
bisexual
bisexuality
B-islet cell
bispecific antibody
bisphosphoglycerate mutase
Bittner
    milk factor, B.
    virus, B.

bivalency
bivalent
Bizzozero's
    cells, B.
    corpuscles, B.
    platelets, B.
black measles
Blackfan-Diamond anemia
blackwater fever
Blakemore-Sengstaken tube
blast
    cell, b.
    cell leukemia, b.
    crisis, b.
    transformation, b.
blastic
    leukemia, b.
blastogenesis
    assay, b.
blastogenic
    factor, b. (BF)
blastomycosis
bleach kit
bleeder
bleeder's disease
bleeding
    diathesis, b.
    time, b. (BT)
Blenoxane
bleomycin
blind
    loop anemia, b.
blinding
blocking
    antibody, b. (BA)
    factors, b.
blood
    anticoagulated b.
    arterial b.
    citrated b.
    cord b.
    defibrinated b.
    laked b.
    laky b.
    occult b.
    peripheral b.

blood *(continued)*
  pooled b.
  sludged b.
  splanchnic b.
  transfused b.
  venous b.
  whole b.
blood agar
  plate, b. (BAP)
blood-air barrier
blood alcohol concentration (BAC)
blood antibody type
blood-aqueous barrier
blood bank
blood-based test
blood bicarbonate
blood-borne
blood-brain barrier (BBB)
blood buffering capacity
blood cell
  casts, b.
blood-cerebral barrier
blood-cerebrospinal fluid barrier
blood chemistry
blood cholesterol
blood clot
  lysis time, b.
blood clotting
  factor, b.
  time, b.
blood coagulation
  factors, b.
    I fibrinogen
    II prothrombin
    III thromboplastin
    IV calcium ions
    V proaccelerin OR accelerator globulin
    VI Factor VI
    VII proconvertin OR serum prothrombin conversin accelerator
    VIII antihemophilic factor OR von Willebrand's factor
    IX plasma thromboplastin component OR Christmas factor

blood *(continued)*
    X Stuart factor OR Stuart-Prower factor
    XI plasma thromboplastin antecedent
    XII Hageman factor
    XIII fibrin stabilizing factor
blood collection
blood component
blood corpuscle
blood count
blood crossmatching
blood crystals
blood culture
blood cytolysate
blood donor
blood doping
blood drawing
blood dust
blood dyscrasia
blood exchange
blood expander
blood extravasation
blood film
blood flow
blood flowmeter
blood fluke
blood fraction
blood gases
blood ghost
blood glucose (bG)
blood granulocyte-specific activity (BGSA)
blood group
  ABO b.
  Auberger b.
  Cartwright b.
  Diego b.
  Dombrock b.
  Duffy b.
  high frequency b.
  I b.
  Kell b.
  Kell-Cellano b.
  Kidd b.
  Lewis b.

blood group *(continued)*
   low frequency b.
   Lutheran b.
   MN b.
   MNSs b.
   P b.
   Rh b.
blood group antigen
blood group chimera
blood grouping serum
blood islands
blood islets
blood levels
blood lipids
blood panel
blood patch
blood perfusion
   monitor, b. (BPM)
   scan, b.
blood picture
blood pigment
blood plasma
blood plate thrombus
blood platelet thrombus
blood platelets
blood plates
blood poisoning
blood pool scan
blood pressure (BP)
   cuff, b.
   monitor, b.
blood products
blood profile
blood pump
blood reservoir
blood sample
blood screening
blood serum
blood shunting
blood smear
blood specimen
blood spill
blood splash
blood substitute
blood sugar
blood test

blood-thymus barrier
blood transfusion
blood type
blood typing
blood urea nitrogen (BUN)
blood vessel
blood volume
blood warmer
blood work
bloodless
   field, b.
   phlebotomy, b.
bloodletting
bloodshot
bloodstream
bloody
   sweat, b.
   weeping, b.
Bloom syndrome
blot test
blotting
blue
   baby, b.
   bloater, b.
Blum's syndrome
B-lymphocyte
   stimulatory factor, B. (BSF)
BMD (bone marrow depression)
B- (Mediterranean) variant
BMG (benign monoclonal gammopathy)
B2MG (beta-2-microglobulin)
B-2 microglobulin
BMY-27857
BMY-40900
body
   Amato b.
   Arnold's b.
   asteroid b.
   Auer b.
   Bence Jones b.
   Bracht-Wachter b.
   brassy b.
   Cabot's ring b.
   Call-Exner b.
   Councilman b.

body *(continued)*
    Cowdry type A intranuclear inclusion b.
    Deetjen's b.
    demilune b.
    Dohle's b.
    Dohle's inclusion b.
    Donovan b.
    Dutcher b.
    Ehrlich's hemoglobinemia b.
    elementary b.
    gamma-Favre b.
    Gamna-Gandy b.
    Gordon's elementary b.
    Guarnieri's b.
    Heinz b.
    Heinz-Ehrlich b.
    Howell's b.
    Howell-Jolly b.
    immune b.
    inclusion b.
    inner b.
    Jolly b.
    jugular b.
    ketone b.
    Lallemand's b.
    Lallemand-Trousseau b.
    Leishman-Donovan b.
    Lipschutz b.
    lyssa b.
    Mott b.
    Negri b.
    Neill-Mooser b.
    Pappenheimer b.
    Paschen b.
    Prowazek's b.
    Prowazek-Greeff b.
    pyknotic b.
    Reilly b.
    Ross' b.
    Russell b.
    Seidelin b.
    Trousseau-Lallemand b.
body defenses
body fluid exchange
body fluids
Boeck's sarcoid
Boivin antigen
Bolivian hemorrhagic fever
bolus
bolused
Bombay phenotype
bombesin GRP immunoreactivity
bone marrow
    aspirate, b.
    aspiration, b.
    biopsy, b.
    cell, b.
    depression, b. (BMD)
    differential count, b.
    pool, b.
    progenitor cell, b.
    suppression, b.
    transplant, b.
boost dose
boosted
booster
    immunization, b.
    response, b.
Bordetella pertussis
Bordet-Gengou phenomenon
Borrelia burgdorferi
Boston exanthem
botulinum toxin
botulinus toxin
botulism
bound
    antigen, b.
    label, b.
    serum iron, b. (BSI)
bovine
    dialyzable leukocyte extract, b.
    gamma globulin, b. (BGG)
    lentovirus, b.
    leukemia virus, b.
    red blood cells, b. (BRBC)
    serum albumin, b. (BSA)
bowel
    perforation, b.
    wall penetration, b.
Boyden chamber
boy-in-a-bubble disease

BP (blood pressure)
BPM (blood perfusion monitor)
brachioproctic eroticism
Bracht-Wachter bodies
branched chain
brassy body
BRBC (bovine red blood cells)
breakbone fever
BRMs (biological response modifiers)
bromelain
Brompton cocktail
bronzed disease
Brunhilde virus
Bruton's agammaglobulinemia
BSA (bovine serum albumin)
BSF (B-lymphocyte stimulating factor)
BSI (bound serum iron)
BSL (biosafety level)
BT (bleeding time)
B-2 lymphoma virus
bubble boy disease
buccal
   mucosa, b.
   smear, b.
Buckley's syndrome
budding forms
Buerger-Grutz disease
buffer
buffering
buffy coat
   smear, b.
buffy-coated cell
bulla (pl. bullae)

bullae (pl. of bulla)
Bullis fever
Buminate
BUN (blood urea nitrogen)
Bunyamwera virus
Bunyaviridae
bunyavirus
Buretrol
Burkitt
   lymphoma, B.
   -like lymphoma, B.
   -type acute lymphoblastic leukemia, B.
burr
   cell, b.
   erythrocyte, b.
bursa of Fabricius
bursitis
burst-forming unit-erythroid (BFU-E)
Buschke-Lowenstein tumor
busulfan (Myleran)
butterfly
   needle, b.
   rash, b.
butyl-DNJ (deoxynojirimycin)
butyl nitrite (popper)
butylated hydroxytoluene (BHT)
Butzler Campylobacter virus
buyer's club
BV-ara-U
B- (Mediterranean) variant
Bwamba virus

Additional entries _____

_____
_____
_____
_____
_____
_____

C

Cabot's ring bodies
cacation
cacatory
Cache valley virus
cachectic
cachectin
cachexia
cadaver
    blood transfusion, c.
    transplant, c.
CADD-PLUS (an intravenous infusion pump)
calcemia
calcified thrombus
Calcimar
calcimeter
calcinosis
calcitonin
calcium pyrophosphate dihydrate (CPPD)
calcivirus
calcoglobulin
California virus
CALLA (common acute lymphoblastic leukemia antigen)
CALLA + T-Ig phenotype
Call-Exner bodies
Calmette's vaccine
Calmette-Guerin bacille (CGB)
CAM (cell adhesion molecule)
cameloid
    anemia, c.
    cell, c.
CAMP
    factor, C.
    test, C.
Campylobacter
    jejuni, C.
campylobacter fetus enteritis
campylobacteriosis
canalized thrombus
canceremia
cancer
    -associated anemia, c.

cancer *(continued)*
    -free white mouse, c. (CFWM)
    -inducing virus, c.
Candida
    albicans, C.
candidal
    arthritis, c.
candidemia
candidiasis
Caner-Decker syndrome
Cannabic
cannabinoid
cannabis
cannabism
Cantell alpha interferon
cantharides
cantharidism
CA-19-9 antigen
CA-125 antigen
capillary
    action, c.
    attraction, c.
    bed, c.
    blood sugar, c. (CBS)
    exchange, c.
    fluid shift, c.
    flow, c.
    fragility, c.
    pores, c.
    pulsation, c.
    refill, c.
Caplan's syndrome
capsaicin
capsular antigen
Carazzi's hematoxylin
carbohemia
carbohemoglobin
carbolfuchsin stain
Carbovir
carboxyhemoglobin
carboxyhemoglobinemia
carboxyhemoglobinuria
carboxymyoglobin

carcinoembryonic antigen (CEA)
cardiogenic shock
cardiolipin
cardioplegia
cardioplegic
CA15-2 RIA
carotenemia
carrier
Carrion's disease
carrisyn
cascade
Caspersson type B cells
Castaneda bottle
castanospermine
Castle's intrinsic factor
castration
    cells, c.
casual sex
cat scratch
    disease, c.
    fever, c.
catabolic
catabolism
catalysis
catalyze
catfish sting
cathemoglobin
cationic proteins
Catu virus
CAVH (continuous arteriovenous hemofiltration)
CA (croup-associated) virus
CBC (complete blood count)
CBCT (community-based clinical trials)
CBG (corticosteroid-binding globulin OR cortisol-binding protein)
C4 binding protein
CBS (capillary blood sugar)
CBV (central OR circulating OR corrected blood volume)
CCA (chick-cell agglutination OR chimpanzee coryza agent)
CCAT (conglutinating complement absorption test)
CCF (crystal-induced chemotactic factor)
CD (cluster of differentiation)

CD4
    cells, C.
    helper cells, C.
    lymphocyte, C.
    receptor, C.
    T-cell, C,
    -IgG, C.
    -Pseudomonas exotoxin, C.
CD4+ cells
CD8
    cells, C.
    lymphocyte, C.
    T-cell, C.
CD8+ cells
CD18 antigen
CDA (congenital dyserythropoietic anemia)
cdA (chlorodeoxyadenosine)
2-cdA (2-chlorodeoxyadenosine)
CDC (Centers for Disease Control)
CDC/AIDS (Centers for Disease Control for Diagnosis of AIDS)
cDNA (complementary DNA)
cDNA clones
CDP (cytidine diphosphate)
CDR (complementarity-determining region)
CEA (carcinoembryonic antigen)
    -Roche assay, C.
    -Tc-99m (ImmuRAID), C.
celibacy
celibate
cell
    Abbe-Zeiss counting c.
    accessory c.
    adherent c.
    adventitial c.
    antigen-presenting c.
    antigen-reactive c.
    antigen-sensitive c.
    Aschoff's c.
    B c.
    balloon c.
    band c.
    basophilic c.
    berry c.

cell *(continued)*
    blast c.
    blood c.
    bone marrow c.
    buffy-coated c.
    burr c.
    cameloid c.
    Caspersson type B c.
    CD4 helper c.
    CD4+ c.
    CD8+ c.
    cell-mediated immunity c.
    committed c.
    contrasuppressor c.
    counting c.
    Custer c.
    cytotoxic T c.
    daughter c.
    dendritic c.
    dendritic epidermal c.
    Dorothy Reed c.
    Downey c.
    eating c.
    effector c.
    emigrated c.
    endothelioid c.
    enterochromaffin c.
    epithelioid c.
    erythroid c.
    Ferratea's c.
    follicular dendritic c.
    foreign body giant c.
    ghost c.
    giant c.
    glitter c.
    grape c.
    hairy c.
    HeLa c.
    helmet c.
    helper c.
    hematopoietic stem c.
    Hodgkin's c.
    homozygous typing c. (HTC)
    Hurthle c.
    hybrid c.
    hybridoma c.

cell *(continued)*
    hyperchromatic c.
    immunologically competent c.
    inclusion c.
    inducer c.
    inflammatory c.
    interdigitating c.
    interfollicular c.
    intracytoplasmic inclusion c.
    juvenile c.
    K c.
    killer c.
    Kuppfer's c.
    L c.
    lacunar c.
    LAK c.
    Langerhans' c.
    Langhans' giant c.
    LE c.
    Leishman's chrome c.
    lepra c.
    littoral c.
    Loevit c.
    Lyl B c.
    lymph c.
    lymphadenoma c.
    lymphoid c.
    lymphokine-activated killer c.
    lymphoreticular c.
    Marchand's c.
    marrow c.
    mast c.
    maturation B c.
    mediator c.
    memory c.
    migratory c.
    mononuclear c.
    Mooser c.
    morular c.
    mother c.
    Mott c.
    mouth c.
    myeloid c.
    myeloma c.
    Nageotte's c.
    natural killer c.

cell *(continued)*
    Neumann's c.
    neutrophilic c.
    NK c.
    nonadherent c.
    nucleated red blood c.
    null c.
    nurse c.
    oat c.
    oat-shaped c.
    packed human blood c.
    packed red blood c.
    perithelial c.
    pessary c.
    phagocytic c.
    plaque-forming c.
    plasma c.
    PNH c.
    polychromatic c.
    polychromatophil c.
    pre-B c.
    pre-T c.
    pus c.
    RA c.
    ragocyte c.
    Raji c.
    red c.
    red blood c.
    Reed c.
    Reed-Sternberg giant c.
    rhagiocrine c.
    Rieder c.
    Rindfleisch's c.
    rod c.
    rosette c.
    Rouget c.
    round c.
    scavenger c.
    segmented c.
    sensitized c.
    Sezary c.
    shadow c.
    sickle c.
    sinusoidal endothelial c.
    smudge c.
    spindle-shaped c.

cell *(continued)*
    spur c.
    stab c.
    staff c.
    stave c.
    stem c.
    Sternberg's giant c.
    Sternberg-Reed c.
    stipple c.
    suppressor c.
    T c.
    T4 c.
    T8 c.
    target c.
    tart c.
    T-cytotoxic c.
    Tdth c.
    Thoma-Zeiss counting c.
    thymic epithelial c.
    thymus-dependent c.
    thymus nurse c.
    Touton giant c.
    T-suppressor c.
    Turk's c.
    veil c.
    veiled c.
    veto c.
    Virchow c.
    von Kupffer's c.
    wandering c.
    Warthin's c.
    Warthin-Finkeldey c.
    white c.
    white blood c.
cell adhesion molecule (CAM)
cell assay test
cell bank
cell blockade
cell-bound antibody
cell color ration
cell count
cell-fixed antibody
cell interaction (CI) genes
cell kinetics
cell leukemia lymphosarcoma
cell lines

cell marker
cell-mediated
   immune response, c.
   immunity, c. (CMI)
   lympholysis, c.
cell membrane
cell proliferation
Cell Saver Haemolite
cell sorter
cell strain
cell-surface marker
Cellano phenotype
celltrifuge
cellular
   adaptation, c.
   immunity, c.
   immunity deficiency syndrome, c. (CIDS)
   immunodeficiency, c.
   rejection, c.
   suppression, c.
cellularity
cellulotoxic
CEM/HIV-1 cell line
Centers for Disease Control (CDC)
centigray (cGy)
centistoke
central
   blood volume, c. (CBV)
   line, c.
   nervous system, c. (CNS)
Centry
cephalhematocele
cephalhematoma
cephalin
   -cholesterol flocculation test, c.
Cephalosporium
   granulomatis, C.
cerebrospinal fluid (CSF)
Cerubidine
ceruloplasmin
Cetus trial
CF (Christmas factor OR complement-fixing OR complement fixation)
   antibody titer, C.
CFA (complement-fixing antibody)

CFIDS (chronic fatigue and immune dysfunction syndrome)
CFT (complement-fixation test)
CFU (colony-forming unit)
CFU-C (colony-forming unit-culture)
CFU-E (colony-forming unit-erythroid)
CFU-eos (colony-forming unit-eosinophil)
CFU-F (colony-forming unit-fibroblast)
CFU-GM (colony-forming unit-granulocyte macrophage)
CFU-L (colony-forming unit-lymphoid)
CFU-M (colony-forming unit-megakaryocyte)
CFU-nm (colony-forming unit-neutrophil monocyte)
CFU-S (colony-forming unit-spleen)
CFWM (cancer-free white mouse)
CGL (chronic granulocytic leukemia)
CGP (circulating granulocyte pool)
cGy (centigray
C'H450 complement
CHA (congenital hypoplastic anemia)
Chaetomium
Chagas' disease
Chagres' virus
chain
   branched c.
   closed c.
   H (heavy) c.
   heavy c.
   J (joining) c.
   joining c.
   kappa c.
   lambda c.
   lateral c.
   light c.
   side c.
chain-initiation codons
chain-termination codons
chain terminator
chaining
chancre
chancroid
Charcot
   arthropathy, C.

Charcot *(continued)*
   -like arthropathy, C.
Charcot-Leyden crystal
checker colony
Chediak-Higashi syndrome
chelates
chelating agent
chelation
chemiluminescence
chemistry
   profile, c.
   values, c.
chemoattractant
chemobiotic
chemoimmunology
chemoreceptor trigger zone (CTZ)
chemoresistance
chemosensitive
chemoserotherapy
chemosmosis
chemotactic
   activity, c.
   factor, c.
chemotactin
chemotaxis
   assay, c.
chemotherapeutic
chemotherapy
Chemstrip MatchMaker blood glucose
   meter
Chenuda virus
chick-cell agglutination (CCA)
chicken fat clot
chickenpox
Chido-Rodgers antigen
chief agglutinin
chikungunya fever virus
chimera
chimerism
chimpanzee coryza agent (CCA)
Chinese
   Compound Q, C.
   cucumber, C.
   trichosanthin, C.
Chiron strip
Chlamydia

Chlamydia *(continued)*
   psittaci, C.
   trachomatis, C.
chlamydial
chlofamine
chlorambucil
chloramphenicol
chloride shift
chlorodeoxyadenosine (cdA)
2-chlorodeoxyadenosine (2-cdA)
chloroleukemia
chloroquine
chlorotic anemia
chlorpromazine
cholera
   toxin, c.
   vaccine, c.
cholesteremia
cholesterinized antigen
cholesterol
   level, c.
   screening, c.
cholesterolemia
Cholybar
chorioretinitis
Christmas
   disease, C.
   factor, C. (CF)
chromatogram
chromatography
chromomere
chromoprotein
chromosomal
   sex, c.
chromosome
   banding, c.
   manipulation, c.
   map, c.
   walking, c.
chromotope sodium
chronic
   fatigue and immune dysfunction syn-
      drome, c. (CFIDS)
   granulocytic leukemia, c. (CGL)
   granulomatous disease, c.

chronic *(continued)*
   inflammatory demyelinating polyradiculoneuropathy, c. (CIDP)
   lymphadenopathy syndrome, c.
   lymphatic leukemia, c. (CLL)
   lymphoblastic leukemia, c. (CLL)
   lymphocytic leukemia, c. (CLL)
   lymphosarcoma leukemia, c. (CLSL)
   monoblastic leukemia, c. (CMoL)
   monocytic leukemia, c. (CMoL)
   myelocytic leukemia, c. (CML)
   myelogenous leukemia, c. (CML)
   myeloid leukemia, c.
chrysotherapy
Churg-Strauss syndrome
Chvostek's
   anemia, C.
   sign, C.
chylomicronemia
chymotrypsin
CI (cell interaction) genes
CIC (circulating immune complexes)
CID (cytomegalic inclusion disease)
cidal
   level, c.
CIDP (chronic inflammatory demyelinating polyradiculoneuropathy)
CIDS (cellular immunity deficiency syndrome)
CIE (countercurrent immunoelectrophoresis)
CIEP (counterimmunoelectrophoresis)
CIF (clonal-inhibiting OR inhibitory factor)
CIg (cytoplasmic immunoglobulin)
ciguatera
ciguatoxin
Cilofungin
C3b inactivator
   accelerator, C.
Cipro (ciprofloxacin)
ciprofloxacin
circulating
   anticoagulants, c.
   antithromboplastin disorder, c.
   atypical lymphocytes, c.

circulating *(continued)*
   blood volume, c. (CBV)
   granulocyte pool, c. (CGP)
   immune complexes, c. (CIC)
   red cells, c.
circulation
   time, c.
circulatory
   collapse, c.
   failure, c.
circumanal
circumscribed scleroma
cisplatin
cis-platinum
citrated plasma
citrate-phosphate-dextrose (CPD)
   adenine, c. (CPDA-l)
citrovorum
   factor, c.
   rescue, c.
CI-898
CK (creatine kinase)
C1 inhibitor
Clara's hematoxylin
Claricid
clarithromycin
Clark-Collip method
clasmatocyte
clasmatocytic
   lymphoma, c.
Class I, II, III antigens
classification of leukemia
   FAB-M1   myeloblastic, with no differentiation
   FAB-M2   myeloblastic, with differentiation
   FAB-M3   promyelocytic
   FAB-M5   monocytic
   FAB-M6   erythroleukemia
clathrin
Clausen's method
clearance
cleavage
   products, c.
Cleveland procedure
Clinacox

clindamycin
CLL (chronic lymphatic OR lymphoblastic OR lymphocytic leukemia)
clofazimine
clonal
    deletion theory, c.
    expansion, c.
    inhibiting factor, c. (CIF)
    inhibitory factor, c. (CIF)
    selection theory, c.
clone
cloned gene
cloning vector
clonogenic
Clorox bleach
    assay, C.
    technique, C.
clonotypic
clostridial toxin
Clostridium
    difficile, C.
    perfringens, C.
clot
    lysis, c.
    lysis time, c. (CLT)
    reaction, c.
    retraction time, c.
clotrimazole
clotting
    enzyme, c.
    factor, c.
    parameters, c.
    study, c.
    time, c.
Clough and Richter's syndrome
CLSL (chronic lymphosarcoma leukemia)
CLT (clot-lysis time)
clubbing
clumped cells
clumping of cells
cluster of differentiation (CD)
CM II virus
CM-5-FU
CMI (cell-mediated immunity)
CMID (cytomegalic inclusion disease)

CML (chronic myelocytic OR myelogenous leukemia OR cell-mediated lympholysis)
CMoL (chronic monoblastic OR monocytic leukemia)
CMP (cytidine monophosphate)
CMV (cytomegalovirus)
    colitis, C.
    hepatitis, C.
    immune globulin, C.
    mononucleosis, C.
    retinitis, C.
    triclonal antibodies, C.
C3NeF (C3 nephritic factor)
C3 nephritis factor (C3NeF)
CNHD (congenital nonspherocytic hemolytic disease)
CNS (central nervous system)
    leukemia, C.
CoA (coenzyme A)
coag (coagulase)
coagglutination
coagula (pl. of coagulum)
coagulability
coagulable
coagulant
coagulase
coagulate
coagulating
    enzyme, c.
    factor, c.
coagulation
    factor, c.
    factor assay, c.
    pathways, c.
    time, c.
coagulative
coagulator
coagulogram
coagulometer
coagulopathy
coagulum (pl. coagula)
CoA-transferase
cobalamin
    adenosyltransferase, c.
cobalt

Cobe double blood pump
cobweb
cocaine
    baby, c.
    metabolites, c.
cocainization
cocainize
cocainomania
co-capping
coccidian protozoan
Coccidioides
    immitis, C.
coccidioidin
coccidioidomycosis
coctoantigen
cocto-immunogen
coctolabile
coctoprecipitin
coctostabile
cocultivation
coculture
codominance
codominant genes
codon
Coe virus
coefficient
coenzyme
    A, c. (CoA)
    Q, c. (CoQ)
coexistent chronic myelogenous leukemia
cofactor
coffee grounds material
COHB (carboxyhemoglobin)
cohesion
cohesive end
Cohn fraction II
cohort
    life table, c.
    study, c.
coital
coitus
co-labeled vitamin B-12
colchicine
cold
    agglutination, c.
    agglutinin, c.

cold *(continued)*
    antibody, c.
    hemagglutinin, c.
    hemolysin test, c.
    -insoluble proteins, c.
    -reacting antibody, c.
    urticaria, c.
coldsore
Cole's hematoxylin
Coley's toxin
colicolitis
colilysin
colitis
collagen
collagenase
collagenolysis
collateral flow
Collison's fluid
Collostat
coloenteritis
colon perforation
colony
colony-forming unit
    -culture, c. (CFU-C)
    -eosinophil, c. (CFU-eos)
    -erythroid, c. (CFU-E)
    -fibroblast, c. (CFU-F)
    -lymphoid, c. (CFU-L)
    -megakaryocyte, c. (CFU-M)
    -neutrophil monocyte, c. (CFU-nm)
    -spleen, c. (CFU-S)
colony-stimulating factor (CSF)
coloproctitis
color index
Colorado tick fever virus
colorectal
colorectitis
colorectum
Colorgene DNA Hybridization Test
Columbia
    blood agar, C.
    -SK virus, C.
Colyonal
combination chemotherapy
combined immunodeficiency
combining site antibody

committed cell
common
    acute lymphoblastic leukemia antigen, c. (CALLA)
    antigen, c.
    cold virus, c.
    variable agammaglobulinemia, c.
    variable hypogammaglobulinemia, c. (CVH)
    variable immunodeficiency, c. (CVI)
communal needle
communicable
community immunity
COMP
compassionate use
compatibility
compensatory polycythemia
competitive bonding
complement
    activation, c.
    assay, c.
    cascade, c.
    deficiency, c.
    -dependent, c.
    deviation, c.
    fixation, c.
    -fixation test, c. (CFT)
    -fixing antibody, c. (CFA)
    fragment, c.
    inactivation, c.
    level, c.
    lysis sensitivity test, c.
    -mediated anaphylaxis, c.
    -mediated cytotoxicity, c.
    receptor, c.
    sequence, c.
    unit, c.
C3 complement receptors
complementarity-determining region (CDR)
complementary
    bases, c.
    DNA, c. (cDNA)
    genes, c.
complementation
complementophil
complete
    antibody, c.
    blood count, c. (CBC)
complotype
compluetic reaction
compound
    leukemia, c.
Compound Q (CoQ)
Compound S (CoS)
ConA (concavalin A)
concavalin A (ConA)
concomitant immunity
condom
condyloma (condylomata)
condylomata
conformation
conformational determinant
congeners
congenital
    agammaglobulinemia, c.
    anemia of newborn, c.
    dyserythropoietic anemia, c. (CDA)
    hypoplastic anemia, c. (CHA)
    immunity, c.
    nonspherocytic hemolytic disease, c. (CNHD)
conglutinating complement absorption test (CCAT)
conglutination
    reaction, c.
conglutinin
conglutinogen
    -activating factor, c. (KAF)
Congo-Crimean hemorrhagic fever virus
conjugated antigen
consanguineous donor
consolidation therapy
constant region gene
constitutional
    hyperbilirubinemia, c.
    thrombopathy, c.
consumption coagulopathy
contact
    activation product, c.
    factor, c.

continuous arteriovenous hemofiltration (CAVH)
contrasuppressor cells
controlled substance
convalescent serum
Cook catheter
cook (person who makes illegal drugs or the process of making them)
cooker (drug paraphernalia)
Cooley's anemia
Coombs' test
cooperator cell
coproantibody
coprohematology
coprolagnia
coprophagous
coprophagy
coprophilia
coproporphyria
coproporphyrin
copulating pouch
copulation
CoQ (coenzyme Q or Compound Q)
coral thrombus
cord
    blood, c.
    pH, c.
core
    antigen, c.
    particles, c.
    protein, c.
Cormed pump
coronavirus
corpuscle
corpuscular
corrected blood volume (CBV)
corticosteroid
    binding globulin, c.- (CBG)
cortisol-binding globulin (CBG)
Cortrosyn
Corynebacterium
    infantisepticum, C
    parvulum, C.
coryzavirus
cothromboplastin
cotinine

co-trimoxazole
cotton wool
    patch, c.
    spot, c.
Coulter counter
Coumadin
coumadinize
Councilman bodies
count
    Addis c.
    Arneth c.
    blood c.
    complete blood c.
    differential c.
    direct platelet c.
    filament-nonfilament c.
    indirect platelet c.
    manual differential c.
    neutrophil lobe c.
    red blood cell c.
    reticulocyte c.
    Schilling blood c.
    staff c.
    white blood cell c.
countercurrent exchanger
    immunoelectrophoresis, c. (CIE)
counterelectrophoresis
counterflow centrifugal elutriation
counterimmunoelectrophoresis (CIEP)
counting
    cell, c.
    plate, c.
covalent bond
Cowdry type A intranuclear inclusion bodies
cowpox
cow's milk
    anemia, c.
    immune globulin, c.
Cox vaccine
coxotuberculosis
coxsackievirus (C virus)
CPD (citrate-phosphate-dextrose)
CPDA-l (citrate-phosphate-dextrose-adenine)
CPF

CPK (creatine phosphokinase)
CPPD (calcium pyrophosphate dihydrate)
C3PA proactivator
crabs
crack
    baby, c.
    cocaine, c.
    house, c.
Crasnitin
C-reactive protein (CRP)
creatine
    kinase, c. (CK)
    phosphokinase, c. (CPK)
creatinemia
creatinine clearance
C3 receptor
C3a receptor
C5a receptor
creeping thrombosis
CREG (cross-reactive group)
crenated erythrocyte
crenation
crenocyte
crenocytosis
crescent
    bodies, c.
    cell anemia, c.
cresyl blue
Crimean hemorrhagic fever
crit (hematocrit)
Crithidia
    lucilliae, C.
Crohn's disease
cromolyn
cross
    -agglutination, c.
    -dresser, c.
    -dressing, c.
    -immunity, c.
    -link, c.
    -matching, c.
    -reacting antibody, c.
    -reacting antigen, c.
    -reaction, c.
    -reactivation, c.
    -reactive group, c. (CREG)

cross *(continued)*
    -reactivity, c.
    -resistance, c.
    -sensitization, c.
crossed immunoelectrophoresis
crossmatch
crossmatching
crossover trial
croup-associated (CA) virus
CRP (C-reactive protein)
cruise
cruiser
cruising
cryocrit value
cryofibrinogen
cryofibrinogenemia
cryogammaglobulin
cryogen
cryogenic
cryoglobulin
cryoglobulinemia
cryopathic hemolytic syndrome
cryoprecipitability
cryoprecipitate
cryoprecipitated antihemophilic factor
cryoprecipitation
cryopreservation
cryopreserved
cryoprotective
cryoprotein
cryostat
crypto (cryptococcosis or cryptosporidiosis)
cryptococcal
    antigen, c.
    meningitis, c.
Cryptococcus
    neoformans, C.
cryptoleukemia
cryptosporidial
cryptosporidiosis
    antibody, c.
Cryptosporidium
    listeria, C.
cryptosporidium immune whey protein
    concentrate

crystal
  violet, c.
  -induced chemotactic factor, c. (CCF)
CS-85
CS-87
CSF (cerebrospinal fluid OR colony-stimulating factor)
CT (clinical trials)
C-terminal constant region
CTL (cytotoxic T-lymphocytes)
CTP (cytidine triphosphate)
C-type retrovirus
CTZ (chemoreceptor trigger zone)
cuffing
culture
  medium, c.
  sensitivity, c. and (C&S)
cultured up
cumulative
  dose, c.
  genes, c.
cunnilinctus
cunnilinguist
cunnilingus
cupping
cupremia
cupric sulfate
curd
currant jelly clot
Curvularia
Cushing's basophilism
Custer cells
cut-off value
cut point
cutaneous anaphylaxis
cutdown
CVH (common variable hypogammaglobulinemia)
CVI (common variable immunodeficiency)
C virus (coxsackievirus)
cyanemia
cyanhematin
cyanhemoglobin
cyanmethemoglobin
cyanmetmyoglobin
cyanocobalamin
cyanosed
cyanosis
cyanotic
cyclobenzaprine
cycloheximide
cylo-oxygenase
cyclophosphamide
cycloserine
cyclosporin A
cyclosporine
cytarabine
cytidine
  deaminase, c.
  diphosphate, c. (CDP)
  monophosphate, c. (CMP)
  triphosphate, c. (CTP)
cytoanalyzer
cytochalasin
  B, c.
cytochemical
cytochemistry
cytochrome
  b5 reductase, c.
  c oxidase, c.
  P-450 reductase, c.
cytocidal
cytocide
cytoclasis
cytoclesis
cytocrit
cytoctic
cytoctony
cytodieresis
cytogenic
  anemia, c.
cytoglomerator
cytoglucopenia
cytoglycopenia
cytoid
cytokalipenia
cytokine
cytologic
  T-lymphocyte, c.
cytolysate
cytolysin

cytolysis
cytolytic
cytomegalic
    inclusion disease, c. (CID or CMID)
cytomegaloviruria
cytomegalovirus (CMV)
cytometer
cytometry
cytomorphology
cytomorphosis
cytopathic
cytopenia
cytophilic
    antibody, c.
cytoplasm
cytoplasmic
    immunoglobulin, c. (CIg)
    inclusion, c.
cytorrhyctes
Cytosar
Cytosar-U

cytosine arabinoside (Ara-C)
cytostasis
cytostatic
cytotactic
cytotaxigen
cytotaxis
cytotoxic
    antibody, c.
    suppressor, c.
    T-cell, c.
    T-lymphocyte, c. (CTL)
cytotoxicity
cytotoxin
cytotrophic
    serum, c.
cytotropic
    antibody, c.
cytotropism
Cytovene
Cytoxan
CyVADIC

Additional entries

D

dacarbazine (Dtic-Dome)
Dacie type II
dactylitis
DAEC (diffuse-adhering E. coli)
DAF (decay-activating factor OR decay antibody-accelerating factor)
DAGT (direct antiglobulin test)
daisy-head colony
Dalacin C
d-ala-peptide T
Dale reaction
Dale-Laidlaw's clotting time
dAMP (deoxyadenosine monophosphate)
danazol
Dane particles
D-antigen
Danysz's phenomenon
dapsone (Avlosulfon)
DAP/TMP (dapsone and trimethoprim)
Daraprim
dark
    blood, d.
    -ground microscopy, d.
darkfield microscopy
dartrous
daughter cell
daunomycin
daunorubicin HCl
Davidsohn's test
dawn phenomenon
Day's factor
D4C
dCMP (deoxycytidine monophosphate)
DCNB (dinitrochlorobenzene)
ddA
DDAVP (desamino-D-arginine vasopressin)
ddC (dideoxycytidine)
ddI (dideoxyinosine)
De Veras Beverage
deallergization
deallergize
deaminase

Dean and Webb titration
DEC (dendritic epidermal cell)
decay
    antibody-accelerating factor, d. (DAF)
    -activating factor, d. (DAF)
decoagulant
decomplementize
D-deficiency factor
Deetjen's bodies
defective virus
defense mechanism
defibrinate
defibrination syndrome
deficiency
    anemia, d.
deficient
definitive erythroblast
degenerative arthritis
deglobulization crisis
deglycerolized red cells
dehydroepiandrosterone (DHEA)
Deitjen's bodies
delayed-type hypersensitivity (DTH)
deletion
Delimmun
delirious
delirium
delta
    agent, d.
    antigen, d.
    hepatitis, d.
demented
dementia
demilune bodies
demyelinated
demyelinating
Dendrid
dendritic
    cell, d.
    epidermal cell, d. (DEC)
dengue
    hemorrhagic fever, d. (DHF)
    virus, d.

dense-deposit disease
dental dam
Denys-Leclef phenomenon
deoxyadenosine
    monophosphate, d. (dAMP)
deoxycytidine
    monophosphate, d. (dCMP)
deoxy-D-glucose
2-deoxy-D-glucose
deoxygenated hemoglobin
deoxygenation
deoxyguanosine monophosphate (dGMP)
deoxyhemoglobin
deoxynojirimycin (butyl-DNJ)
deoxyribonuclease (DNase)
deoxyribonucleic acid (DNA)
deoxythymidine monophosphate (dTMP)
deoxyuridine monophosphate (dUMP)
depressed response
derepressed genes
dermatitis
    herpetiformis, d.
dermatomal herpes zoster
dermatome
dermatomyositis
dermatonecrotic toxin
Dermatophagoides
    farinae, D.
    pteronyssinus, D.
dermatophyton
dermatophytosis
dermographia
desamino-D-arginine vasopressin
    (DDAVP)
desciclovir
desensitization
desensitize
desetope
desexualize
deshydremia
designer drugs
despeciate
despeciated serum
despeciation
despecification
determinant

determinant *(continued)*
    antigenic d.
    conformational d.
    hidden d.
    immunogenic d.
    isoallotypic d.
    isotypic d.
    Kern's isotypic d.
    Km alloptyic d.
    Mcg isotypic d.
    Oz isotypic d.
    sequential d.
DEV (duck embryo vaccine)
dextran sulfate
Dextrarine
Dexulate
DFA (direct fluorescent antibody)
DFMO (difluoromethylornithine)
DGI (disseminated gonococcal infection)
dGMP (deoxyguanosine monophosphate
    OR deoxyguanosine phosphate)
DHE (dihematoporphyrin ether)
DHEA (dehydroepiandrosterone)
DHF (dengue hemorrhagic fever)
DHL (diffuse histiocytic lymphoma)
DHPG (dihydroxypropoxymethylguan-
    ine)
diagnostic diphtheria toxin
dialysance
dialysate
dialysis
    acidosis, d.
    dementia, d.
    disequilibrium, d.
dialyzable
dialyze
dialyzed iron
dialyzer
Diamond-Blackfan anemia
diapedesis
diarrhea
diarrheal
Diascan
diatheses (pl. of diathesis)
diathesis (pl. diatheses)
diathetic

DIC (disseminated or diffuse intravascular coagulation)
Dick
   method, D.
   test, D.
   toxin, D.
diclazuril
Dicopac
dicumarol
didanosine
dideoxycytidine (ddC)
dideoxyinosine (ddI)
didhydrothymidine
Diego antigen
diethylcarbamazine
diethyldithiocarbamate (DTC)
diff (differential)
differential
   agglutination titer, d.
   count, d.
differentiation antigens
diffuse
   histiocytic lymphoma, d. (DHL)
   intravascular coagulation, d. (DIC)
   pigmented villonodular synovitis, d. (DPVNS)
   undifferentiated non-Hodgkin's lymphoma, d. (DUNHL)
   well-differentiated lymphocytic lymphoma, d. (DWDL)
   -adhering E. coli, d. (DAEC)
diffusion factor
Diflucan
difluoromethylornithine (DFMO)
diGugliemo's disease
dihematoporphyrin ether (DHE)
dihydrotestosterone
dihydroxypropoxymethylguanine (DHPG)
dildo
DILE (drug-induced lupus erythematosus)
dilution
   anemia, d.
   -filtration technique, d.
dilutional hyponatremia
dimer

dimethylsulfoxide (DMSO)
dimorphic anemia
DIMP
Dinamap
dinitrochlorobenzene (DNCB)
dinitrophenol
dione
diphenylhydantoin
diphtheria
   antitoxin, d.
   -tetanus, d. (DT)
   toxin, d.
   toxoid, d.
diphtheriaphor
diphtheroid
direct
   agglutination test, d.
   antiglobulin test, d. (DAGT)
   conjugate immunoperoxidase, d.
   Coombs' test, d.
   fluorescent antibody, d. (DFA)
   transfusion, d.
discoid lupus erythematosus (DLE)
disease-modifying antirheumatic drugs (DMARDs)
disequilibrium
disseminated
   candidiasis, d.
   cytomegalovirus, d.
   gonococcal infection, d. (DGI)
   herpes zoster, d.
   intravascular coagulation, d. (DIC)
   lupus erythematosus, d. (DLE)
   Mycobacterium avium complex, d. (DMAC)
dissemination
dissociation constant
distal symmetric peripheral neuropathy (DSPN)
disulfide
   bond bridge, d.
dizotization
DLE (discoid OR disseminated lupus erythematosus)
DMAC (disseminated Mycobacterium avium complex)

DMARDs (disease-modifying antirheumatic drugs)
Dmax
DMSO (dimethylsulfoxide)
DNA (deoxyribonucleic acid)
    chain terminator, D.
    deletion, D.
    footprinting, D.
    histogram, D.
    histone, D.
    lesion, D.
    library, D.
    ligase, D.
    nucleotidylexotransferase, D.
    -ploidy, D.
    polymerase, D.
    probe test, D.
    reassociation, D.
    replication, D.
    restriction enzymes, D.
    sequence, D.
    sequencing, D.
    synthesis, D.
    template, D.
    transfection assay, D.
    virus, D.
DNase (deoxyribonuclease)
    test agar, D.
DNCB (dinitrochlorobenzene)
DNJ (N-butyl-deoxynojirimycin)
Dohle
    bodies, D.
    inclusion bodies, D.
Dolophine
dominance
dominant gene
Donath-Landsteiner
    antibody, D.
    phenomenon, D.
donee
donor
    blood, d.
    marrow, d.
    -specific transfusion, d. (DST)
Donovan bodies
doper

doping
Dorothy Reed cells
dose
    level, d.
    tolerance, d.
double
    -blind study, d.
    diffusion, d.
    minutes, d.
    stranded DNA, d.- (dsDNA)
    stranded RNA, d.- (dsRNA)
dounce glass homogenizer
Dow hollow fiber dialyzer
Downey
    cells, D.
    -type lymphocyte, D.
downgrading reaction
doxorubicin
doxycycline
D-penicillamine
DP-AZT
DPVNS (diffuse pigmented villonodular synovitis)
Drabkin's solution
drag
drepanocyte
drepanocytemia
drepanocytic
    anemia, d.
drepanocytosis
Dresbach's syndrome
dronabinol
droplet infection
drug
    abuse, d.
    abuser, d.
    addict, d.
    -addicted, d.
    addiction, d.
    baby, d.
    dependence, d.
    -dependent, d.
drug-induced
    immune hemolytic anemia, d.
    lupus erythematosus, d. (DILE)
    thrombocytopenia, d.

44 drug lab

drug lab
drug overdose
drug paraphernalia
drug-resistant
drug withdrawal
drugfast
dsDNA (double-stranded DNA)
DSPN (distal symmetric peripheral neuropathy)
dsRNA (double-stranded RNA)
DST (donor-specific transfusion)
D4T
DT (diphtheria/tetanus)
    vaccine, D.
DTC (diethyldithiocarbamate)
DTH (delayed-type hypersensitivity)
Dtic-Dome (dacarbazine)
dTMP (deoxythymidine monophosphate)
DTP (diphtheria/tetanus/pertussis)
    vaccine, D.
dualistic theory
Dubin-Johnson phenomenon
duck
    embryo vaccine, d. (DEV)
    virus hepatitis yolk antibody, d.
Ducrey's bacillus
Duffy
    antibody, D.
    antigen, D.
    blood group, D.
    system, D.
Duke bleeding time
Dukes' classification
Dumdum fever
dUMP (deoxyridine monophosphate OR deoxyridine phosphate)
Duncan's syndrome
DUNHL (diffuse undifferentiated non-Hodgkin's lymphoma)
Dunnet's test
duovirus
DuPont ELISA assay
Duran-Reynals factor
Duret hemorrhage
dust-borne
Dutcher body
DVPL-ASP protocol
DWDL (diffuse well-differentiated lymphocytic lymphoma)
dye reduction spot test
dyscrasia
dyscratic
dysentery
    toxin, d.
dyserythropoiesis
dyserythropoietic
    congenital anemia, d.
dysfibrinogenemia
dysgammaglobulinemia
dysglobulinemia
dysglycemia
dyshematopoiesis
dyshematopoietic
dyslipoproteinemia
dysmyelopoiesis
dysmyelopoietic
    syndrome, d.
dysphagia
dyspoiesis
dyspoietic
dysproteinemia
dysprothrombinemia
D-xylose absorption

Additional entries

E

EA (erythrocyte and antibody)
   rosette, E.
EAC (erythrocyte, antibody, and complement)
   rosette, E.
EACA (epsilon-aminocaproic acid)
EAE (experimental allergic encephalomyelitis)
EAHLG (equine antihuman lymphoblast globulin)
EAHLS (equine antihuman lymphoblast serum)
E antigen
Earle's salts
early erythroblast
easy bruisability
eating cells
Eaton agent
EBL (erythroblastic leukemia)
EBNA (Epstein-Barr nuclear antigen)
Ebola virus
Ebola-Marburg virus
EBV (Epstein-Barr virus)
   antibody, E.
   genomic sequences, E.
ECBO (enteric cytopathogenic bovine orphan)
   virus, E.
ECBV (effective circulating blood volume)
ECC (extracorporeal circulation)
ecchymosis
ecchymotic
ECDO (enteric cytopathogenic dog orphan)
   virus, E.
ECF (eosinophil chemotactic factor OR effective capillary flow)
ECF-A (eosinophil chemotactic factor of anaphylaxis)
ECFV (extracellular fluid volume)
echinocandin
Echinococcus
ECHO (enteric cytopathic human orphan)
   1 virus, E.
   28 virus, E.
echovirus
   28, e.
ECIB (extracorporeal irradiation of blood)
ECIL (extracorporeal irradiation of lymph)
eclampsia
eclamptic
eclamptogenic
ECLT (euglobulin clot lysis time)
ECM (extracellular matrix) protein
ECMO (enteric cytopathogenic monkey orphan or extracorporeal membrane oxygenator)
   virus, E.
E. coli (Escherichia coli)
ecologic fallacy
ECS (extracellular-like, calcium-free solution)
ECSO (enteric cytopathogenic swine orphan)
   virus, E.
ECT (euglobulin clot test)
ecthyma
ecthymiform
ectoantigen
ectopic
   ACTH syndrome, e.
   hypercalcemia syndrome, e.
eczema
eczematous
edathamil
Edelmann's
   anemia, E.
   cell, E.
EDTA (ethylenediaminetetraacetic acid)
effective
   capillary flow, e. (ECF)
   circulating blood volume, e. (ECBV)
   oxygen transport, e. (EOT)
   renal blood flow, e. (ERBF)

effector cells
effeminate
effemination
efficacious
efficacy
eflornithine (DFMO)
Efudex
egg lecithin lipids
EggsAct
EGOT (erythrocyte glutamic oxaloacetic transaminase)
EHEC (enterohemorrhagic E. coli)
Ehlers-Danlos syndrome
Ehrlich's
   hemoglobinemia bodies, E.
   side chain theory, E.
   unit, E.
Ehrlichia
   canis, E.
ehrlichosis
EIA (enzyme immunoassay)
Eichhorst's corpuscles
eicosanoid
eicosapentaenoic acid (EPA)
EID (electroimmunodiffusion)
EIEC (enteroinvasive E. coli)
EIT (erythrocyte iron turnover)
ejaculate
ejaculation
ejaculatory
EL1020
El Tor vibrios
elastometer catheter
electrodialysis
electroejaculation
electroimmunoassay
electroimmunodiffusion (EID)
electrolyte
   balance, e.
   imbalance, e.
electronegative element
electronmicrography
electron-microscopic
electro-osmosis
electropathology
electropherogram
electrophoregram
electrophoresed
electrophoresis
electrophoretic
electrophoretogram
electroporation
electropositive element
electroradioimmunoassay (ERIA)
electrotransfer test
elementary bodies
ELIEDA (enzyme-linked immunoelectrodiffusion assay)
ELISA (enzyme-linked immunosorbent assay)
elliptocytary
   anemia, e.
elliptocyte
elliptocytosis
elliptocytotic
   anemia, e.
elongation factor
Elspar
ELT (euglobulin lysis time)
EL-10 (DHEA)
eluate
eluent
Elutek
elution
elutriate
elutriation
EM (erythema migrans)
emasculation
Embden-Meyerhof pathway
emboli (pl. of embolus)
embolism
embolization
embolus (pl. emboli)
embryogenesis
embryonal leukemia
EMF (eosinophil OR erythrocyte maturation factor)
emigrated cell
emigration
   white cells, e. of
Eminase (anistreplase)
emiocytosis

EMIT (enzyme-multiplied immunoassay technique)
emperic
emperipolesis
ENA (extractable nuclear antigen)
enanthem
ENANB (enterically-transmitted non-A, non-B) hepatitis
enanthesis
encephalitis
Encephalitozoon
   hellem, E.
encephalomyelitis
encephalopathy
encode
endemic
endocarditis
endocrinologic
   sex, e.
endocrinology
endocytosis
endodeoxyribonuclease
endogenous antigen
endoglobular
Endolimax
   nana, E.
endolysin
endonuclease
endopeptidase
endoribonuclease
endorphin
endosmosis
endosmotic
endothelioid cells
endotheliolytic serum
endotoxemia
endotoxicosis
endotoxin
Endoxan
enema
Engel's alkalinity
Engerix-B
enhancing antibody
ENP (extractable nucleoprotein)
Ensure Plus
Entamoeba

Entamoeba *(continued)*
   histolytica, E.
enteral
   nutrition, e.
enteric
   cytopathic human orphan, e. (ECHO)
   cytopathogenic dog orphan, e. (ECDO)
   cytopathogenic monkey orphan, e. (ECMO)
   cytopathogenic swine orphan, e. (ECSO)
   orphan virus, e.
   pathogen, e.
   virus, e.
enterically-transmitted non-A, non-B (ENANB) hepatitis
enteritis
Enterobacter
   aerogenes, E.
   agglomerans, E.
   cloacae, E.
   gergoviae, E.
   liquefaciens, E.
   vermicularis, E.
enterochromaffin cells
enteroclysis
enterococcemia
enterococci (pl. of enterococcus)
enterococcus (pl. enterococci)
enterocolitis
enterohemorrhagic E. coli (EHEC)
enteroinvasive E. coli (EIEC)
enteropathic arthritis
enteropathogenic E. coli (EPEC)
enteropathy
enterorrhagia
enterorrhea
enterorrhexis
enteroscope
enterosepsis
enterospasm
enterostaxis
enterotoxemia
enterotoxigenic E. coli (ETEC)
enterotoxin

enterovirus
entomopox virus
env gene (envelope gene)
Envacor test
envelope
    gene, e.
    protein, e.
environmental antigen
enzymatic
    debridement, e.
    gene amplification, e.
enzyme
    immunoassay, e. (EIA)
enzyme-linked
    antibody test, e.
    immunoelectrodiffusion assay, e. (ELIEDA)
    immunoelectrotransfer, e.
    immunosorbent assay, e.
enzyme-multiplied
    immunoassay technique, e. (EMIT)
enzymopathy
enzymopenia
Eos (eosinophils)
eosin
eosinocyte
eosinopenia
eosinophil
    chemotactic factor, e. (ECF)
    chemotactic factor of anaphylaxis, e. (ECF-A)
    leukocytic infiltrate, e.
    maturation factor, e. (EMF)
    stimulation promoter, e. (ESP)
eosinophilia
eosinophilic
    erythroblast, e.
    exudates, e.
    index, e.
    leukemia, e.
    leukocytes, e.
    leukocytosis, e.
    lung, e.
    series, e.
eosinophilopoietin
eosinophilosis

eosinophilotactic
eosinophilous
eosinophils (Eos)
eosinophiluria
eosinotactic
EOT (effective oxygen transport)
EPA (eicosapentaenoic acid)
EPEC (enteropathogenic E. coli)
EPIblot HIV Western blot test
epidemic
    keratoconjunctivitis virus, e.
    typhus fever vaccine, e.
epidemiologic
epidemiologist
epidemiology
epidermolysis
    bullosa, e.
epinephrine
epinephrinemia
epipodophyllotoxin
epistasis
epistatic
epistaxis
epithelial thymic-activating factor (ETAF)
epithelioid cells
epitope
EPO (erythropoietin)
epoetin alfa
Epogen
EPP (erythropoietic protoporphyria)
Eprex
epsilon
    chain, e.
    -aminocaproic acid, e. (EACA)
Epstein's method
Epstein-Barr
    nuclear antigen, E. (EBNA)
    virus, E. (EBV)
equilibratory
equilibrium
    constant, e.
    dialysis, e.
equine
    antihuman lymphoblast globulin, e. (EAHLG)

equine *(continued)*
    antihuman lymphoblast serum, e. (EAHLS)
    encephalomyelitis virus, e.
ERBF (effective renal blood flow)
ERC (erythropoietin-responsive cell)
erection
ERIA (electroradioimmunoassay)
E rosette
    assay, E.
    formation, E.
    receptor, E.
erosive arthritis
erotic
eroticism
eroticize
erotism
erotize
erotogenesis
erotogenic
erotomania
erotopathy
erotophobia
ERP (estrogen receptor protein)
Erpalfa
Erwinase
erwinia L-asparaginase
erythema
    migrans, e. (EM)
erythremia
erythemic
    myelosis, e.
erythroblast
    acidophilic e.
    basophilic e.
    definitive e.
    early e.
    eosinophilic e.
    orthochromatic e.
    oxyphilic e.
    polychromatic e.
    primitive e.
erythroblastemia
erythroblastic
    anemia of childhood, e.
    leukemia, e. (EBL)

erythroblastoma
erythroblastomatosis
erythroblastopenia
erythroblastosis
    fetalis, e.
    neonatorum, e.
erythroblastosis virus
erythroblastotic
erythrochromia
erythroclasis
erythroclast
erythroclastic
erythrocytapheresis
erythrocyte
    achromic e.
    basophilic e.
    burr e.
    crenated e.
    hypochromic e.
    immature e.
    Mexican hat e.
    normochromic e.
    nucleated e.
    orthochromic e.
    polychromatic e.
    polychromatophilic e.
    target e.
erythrocyte antibody (EA)
erythrocyte, antibody and complement (EAC)
erythrocyte autosensitization
erythrocyte fragility
erythrocyte glutamic oxaloacetic transaminase (EGOT)
erythrocyte iron turnover (EIT)
erythrocyte mass
erythrocyte maturation factor (EMF)
erythrocyte mosaicism
erythrocyte protoporphyrin test
erythrocyte sedimentation rate (ESR)
erythrocyte-sensitizing substance (ESS)
erythrocythemia
erythrocytic
    marrow, e.
    series, e.
erythrocytoblast

erythrocytolysin
erythrocytolysis
erythrocytometer
erythrocytometry
erythrocytoopsonin
erythrocytopenia
erythrocytophagous
erythrocytophagy
erythrocytopoiesis
erythrocytorrhexis
erythrocytoschisis
erythrocytosis
   megalosplenica, e.
erythrocyturia
erythrodegenerative
erythroderma
erythrogenesis
   imperfecta. e.
erythrogenic
   toxin, e.
erythroid
   cells, e.
   hyperplasia, e.
   hypoplasia, e.
erythrokatalysis
erythrokinetics
erythroleukemia
erythroleukoblastosis
erythroleukosis
erythroleukothrombocythemia
erythrolysin
erythrolysis
erythrometer
erythrometry
erythromyeloblastic
   leukemia, e.
erythron
erythroneocytosis
erythronoclastic
erythronormoblastic anemia
erythroparasite
erythropathy
erythropenia
erythrophage
erythrophagia
erythrophagocytic

erythrophagocytic *(continued)*
   lymphohistiocytosis, e.
erythrophagocytosis
erythrophagous
erythrophobia
erythrophthisis
erythroplakia
erythroplasia
   Queyrat, e. of
erythropoiesis
erythropoietic
   porphyria, e.
   protoporphyria, e. (EPP)
   stimulating factor, e. (ESF)
   uroporphyrin, e.
erythropoietin (EPO)
   responsive cell, e.- (ERC)
erythropyknosis
erythrorrhexis
erythrosedimentation
erythrosis
erythrostasis
erythrotoxin
erythuria
escape mechanisms
Escherichia coli (E. coli)
ES-D (esterase-D)
ESF (erythropoietic stimulating factor)
Esmarch bandage
ESP (eosinophil stimulation promoter)
ESR (erythrocyte sedimentation rate)
ESS (erythrocyte-sensitizing substance)
essential
   anemia, e.
   thrombocytosis, e.
esterapenia
esterase-D (ES-D)
esterified estrogens
estradiol
Estren-Damashek anemia
estriol
estrogen
   receptor, e.
   receptor protein, e. (ERP)
   withdrawal bleeding, e.
estrogenic

estrogenicity
estrogenous
estrostilben
ETAF (epithelial thymic-activating factor)
ETEC (enterotoxigenic E. coli)
ethambutol
ethanol gelation test
ethanolism
ethionamide
ethylenediaminetetraacetic acid (EDTA)
etoposide (VP-16)
ETR
eucapnia
eudiemorrhysis
Euglena
    gracilis, E.
euglobulin
    clot lysis time, e. (ECLT)
    clot test, e. (ECT)
    lysis test, e.
    lysis time, e. (ELT)
euglycemia
Eulexin
eunuch
eunuchism
eunuchoid
eunuchoidism
European
    Kaposi's sarcoma, E.
    mistletoe, E.
euthymic
Evans
    blue dye, E.
    staging system, E.
    syndrome, E.
eviration
ExacTec meter
exania
exanthem
exanthema (pl. exanthemata)
exanthemata (pl. of exanthema)
exanthematous
    disease virus, e.
excess antigen
exchange transfusion
exchanger

excitometabolic
exclusion criteria
excrement
excremential absorption
excrementitious
excreta
excystation
exemia
exoantigen
exocolitis
exocrine
exocytosis
exodeoxyribonuclease
exoenzyme
exoerythrocytic plasmodium
exogenous
    antigen cell-bound antibody reaction, e.
    antigen-circulating antibody reaction, e.
    hemosiderosis, e.
exonuclease
exopeptidase
exoribonuclease
exosmosis
exotoxin
expanded
    access, e.
    plasma, e.
experimental allergic encephalomyelitis (EAE)
exsanguinate
exsanguination
    transfusion, e.
exsanguine
exsanguinotransfusion
extracellular
    fluid volume, e. (ECFV)
    matrix (ECM) protein, e.
    toxin, e.
extracorporeal
    circulation, e. (ECC)
    irradiation of blood, e. (ECIB)
    irradiation of lymph, e. (ECIL)
    membrane oxygenator, e. (ECMO)
    photopheresis, e.

extractable
    nuclear antigen, e. (ENA)
    nuclear protein, e. (ENP)
extramedullary
    erythropoiesis, e.
    hematopoiesis, e.
    megakaryocytopoiesis, e.
extrapolate

extrapolation
extravasation
extrinsic
    clotting reaction, e.
    factor, e.
    pathway, e.
ex vivo

Additional entries

F

FA (fluorescent antibody)
Fab (fragment, antigen-binding)
   fragment, F.
   region, F.
FAB (French/American/British) classification of leukemia
Faber's
   anemia, F.
   syndrome, F.
fabism
Facb (fragment, antigen-and-complement-binding)
FACS (fluorescence-activated cell sorter)
FACScan
facteur thymique serique
factor
   A, f.
   accelerator f.
   activation f.
   albumin autoagglutinating f.
   allogeneic effect f.
   angiogenesis f.
   antianemia f.
   antigen-specific T-cell helper f.
   antigen-specific T-cell suppressor f.
   antihemophilic f. A
   antihemophilic f. B
   antihemophilic f. C
   antihemorrhagic f.
   antinuclear f. (ANF)
   anti-pernicious anemia f.
   antiscorbutic f.
   B, f.
   basophil chemotactic f. (BCF)
   B cell differentiation f. (BCDF)
   B cell growth f. (BCGF)
   Bittner milk f.
   blastogenic f. (BF)
   B-lymphocyte stimulatory f. (BSF)
   C3 nephritic f. (C3 NeF)
   CAMP f.
   Castle's f.
   chemotactic f.

factor *(continued)*
   Christmas f.
   citrovorum f.
   clonal inhibitory f. (CIF)
   cloning inhibitory f. (CIF)
   coagulation f.
   colony-stimulating f. (CSF)
   conglutinogen-activating f. (KAF)
   contact f.
   cryoprecipitated antihemophilic f
   crystal-induced chemotactic f. (CCF)
   D, f.
   D deficiency f.
   Day's f.
   decay-activating f. (DAF)
   diffusion f.
   Duran-Reynals f.
   elongation f.
   eluate f.
   eosinophil chemotactic f. (ECF)
   eosinophil chemotactic f. of anaphylaxis (ECF-A)
   epithelial thymic-activating f.
   erythrocyte maturation f. (EMF)
   erythropoietic stimulating f. (ESF)
   extrinsic f.
   fibrin stabilizing f.
   Fitzgerald f.
   Fletcher f.
   glass f.
   glucose tolerance f.
   growth hormone releasing f. (GH-RF)
   growth inhibitory f.
   H, f.
   Hageman f. (HF)
   H deficiency f.
   hepatocyte stimulating f.
   high-molecular-weight neutrophil chemotactic f. (HMN-NCF)
   histamine-releasing f.
   human antihemophilic f.
   hydrazine-sensitive f. (HSF)
   hyperglycemic-glycogenolytic f.

factor *(continued)*
  I deficiency f.
  immunoglobulin-binding f. (IBF)
  inhibiting f.
  initiation f.
  insulin-like growth f. (IGF)
  intrinsic f.
  labile f.
  Lactobacillus casei f.
  Lactobacillus lactis Dorner f.
  Laki-Lorand f.
  LE f.
  leukocyte inhibitory f. (LIF)
  liver Lactobacillus casei f.
  LLD f.
  lymph node permeability f. (LNPF)
  lymphocyte-activating f. (LAF)
  lymphocyte blastogenic f. (LBF)
  lymphocyte mitogenic f. (LMF)
  lymphocyte-transforming f. (LTF)
  lysogenic f.
  macrophage-activating f. (MAF)
  macrophage chemotactic f. (MCF)
  macrophage cytotoxic f.
  macrophage-derived growth f.
  macrophage inhibitory f. (MIF)
  migration inhibitory f.
  milk f.
  mitogenic f.
  mouse mammary tumor f.
  nephritic f.
  neutrophil chemotactic f. (NCF)
  osteoclast-activating f. (OAF)
  P, f.
  Passovoy f.
  platelet f.
  platelet-activating f. (PAF)
  platelet-derived growth f.
  Prower f.
  recruitment f.
  releasing f.
  resistance transfer f.
  resistance-inducing f.
  Rh f.
  Rhesus f.
  rheumatoid f. (RF)

factor *(continued)*
  risk f.
  Simon's septic f.
  skin reactive f. (SRF)
  specific macrophage-arming f. (SMAF)
  stable f.
  Stuart f.
  Stuart-Prower f.
  T-cell growth f.
  thymus-replacing f.
  thyrotropin-releasing f. (TRF)
  transfer f. (TF)
  tumor necrosis f. (NTF)
  V f.
  von Willebrand's f.
  Wills f.
  X f.
factor I   (fibrinogen)
factor II   (prothrombin)
factor III   (multimer assay)
Factor III   (multimer assay)
factor IV   (calcium)
factor V   (proaccelerin)
factor VI   (Factor VI)
factor VII   (serum prothrombin conversion accelerator)
factor VIII   (antihemophilic factor)
factor IX   (plasma thromboplastin)
factor X   (Stuart-Prower factor)
factor XI   (plasma thromboplastin antecedent)
factor XII   (Hageman factor)
factor XIII   (fibrin-stabilizing factor)
Factorate
FAD (flavin adenine dinucleotide)
FADF (fluorescent antibody darkfield)
Fahreus' method
FAIDS (feline AIDS)
false-negative
false-positive
FAMA (fluorescent antibody against membrane antigen)
familial
  erythroblastic anemia, f.

familial *(continued)*
    erythrophagocytic lymphohistiocytosis, f. (FEL)
    immunity, f.
    Mediterranean fever, f. (FMF)
    megaloblastic anemia, f.
    periodic paralysis, f.
FANA (fluorescent antinuclear antibody)
Fanasil
Fanconi's anemia
Fansidar
Far East hemorrhagic fever
Farr test
fast hemoglobin
fasting
    blood sugar, f. (FBS)
    plasma glucose, f. (FPG)
    profile, f.
FAT (fluorescent antibody test)
fatigue toxin
fatty
    acids, f.
    series, f.
FAV (feline ataxia virus)
favism
FBP (fibrinogen breakdown products)
FBS (fasting blood sugar)
Fc
    portion, F.
    receptor, F.
FCA (ferritin-conjugated antibody)
FDP (fibrin degradation product)
Fe (iron)
febrile
    agglutination test, f.
    antigen, f.
    pleiomorphic anemia, f.
fecal
    fat quantitation, f.
feces
FECP (free erythrocyte coproporphyria or coproporphyrin))
FEL (familial erythrophagocytic lymphohistiocytosis)
feline
    AIDS, f. (FAIDS)

feline *(continued)*
    ataxia virus, f. (FAV)
    leukemia virus, f. (FeLV)
    oncornavirus-associated cell membrane antigen, f. (FOCMA)
fellatio
Felton's
    phenomenon, F.
    syndrome, F.
    unit, F.
Felty's syndrome
FeLV (feline leukemia virus)
female pseudohermaphroditism
feminism
feminization
feminizing testes syndrome
femtoliter (fL)
Fenwick's disease
Feostat
FEPP (free erythrocyte protoporphyrin)
Fergon
fermentemia
Fero-Gradumet
Ferrata's cell
ferrated
ferrihemoglobin
ferritin
    -conjugated antibody, f. (FCA)
    -coupled antibody, f.
ferrochelatase
ferroflocculation
ferrohemoglobin
ferrokinetics
ferropexia
ferropexin
ferroprotein
ferrotherapy
ferrous
    fumarate, f.
    gluconate, f.
    lactate, f.
    sulfate, f.
ferroxidase
ferrum
fetal hemoglobin
fetish

fetishism
fetishist
fetoglobin
fetomaternal transfusion
fetoplacental blood
fever
    blister, f.
    unknown origin, f. of (FUO)
F factor
FFP (fresh frozen plasma)
Fi test (fibrinogen test)
FIA (fluorescent immunoassay OR
    fluoroimmunoassay)
FIAC (fiacitabine)
fiacitabine (FIAC)
fialuridine (FIAU)
FIAU (fialuridine)
Fibonacci search scheme
fibremia
fibrin
    degradation product, f. (FDP)
    monomer, f.
    polymer, f.
    split products, f.
    -stabilizing factor, f.
    titer test, f.
fibrinase
fibrinocellular
fibrinogen
    breakdown products, f. (FBP)
    split products, f. (FSP)
fibrinogenase
fibrinogenemia
fibrinogenesis
fibrinogenic
fibrinogenolysis
fibrinogenolytic
fibrinogenopenia
fibrinogenopenic
fibrinogenous
fibrinoid
fibrinokinase
fibrinolysin
fibrinolysis
fibrinolytic
    split products, f. (FSP)

fibrinopenia
fibrinopeptide
fibrinoplastin
fibrinoplatelet
fibrinopurulent
fibrinorrhea
fibrinoscopy
fibrinosis
fibrinous
fibrinuria
fibroblast
fibronectin
field inversion gel electrophoresis (FIGE)
Fiessinger-Leroy syndrome
Fiessinger-Leroy-Reiter syndrome
fifth disease
FIGE (field inversion gel electrophoresis)
filament-nonfilament count
filamentous
    hemoglobin, f.
filariform larvae
Filatori's disease
filopressure
filter
    replacement fluid, f. (FRF)
filterable virus
filtrable virus
filtrate
filtration capacity
fine-needle aspiration biopsy (FNAB)
finger cot
fingerpoke blood sample
fingerprinting
fingerstick blood sample
first-set
    phenomenon, f.
    rejection, f.
fish
    poisoning, f.
    tapeworm disease, f.
Fisher's exact test
Fisher-Race theory
Fisk and Subbarow's method
Fisoneb nebulizer
Fisons nebulizer
fisting

FITC (fluorescein isocyanate)
Fitzgerald factor
fixation
fixed
    blood film, f.
    tissue section, f.
    virus, f.
FK-506
fL (femtoliter)
flagellantism
flagellar
    agglutinin, f.
    antigen, f.
flagellate
flagellation
flare
flattening filter
flavin adenine dinucleotide (FAD)
flavivirus
FLC (Friend leukemia cells)
fleam
Fletcher factor
Flexner-Wintersteiner rosettes
flocculation
floccule
flocculi (pl. of flocculus)
flocculoreaction
flocculus (pl. flocculi)
floor of mouth
flora
flow
    cytometry, f.
    tract, f.
flowmeter
floxuridine (FUdR)
FLT (fluorodeoxythymidine)
flu (influenza)
Fluax
fluconazole
flucytosine
Fludara
fluid
    balance, f.
    exchange, f.
    overload, f.
flu-like syndrome

Fluogen
fluoresce
fluorescein
    conjugated monoclonal antibody, f.
    isocyanate, f. (FITC)
fluorescence
    -activated cell sorter, f. (FACS)
    enhancement, f.
    quenching, f.
fluorescent
    antibody, f. (FA)
    antibody against membrane antigen, f. (FAMA)
    antibody darkfield, f. (FADF)
    antibody technique, f.
    antibody test, f. (FAT)
    antinuclear antibody, f. (FANA)
    auramine-rhodamine stain, f.
    spot test, f.
    treponemal antibody, f. (FTA)
    treponemal antibody-absorption test for syphilis, f. (FTA-ABS)
fluoro-ddC
fluorodeoxythymidine (FLT)
fluorodeoxyuridine (FUdR)
fluorography
fluoroimmunoassay (FIA)
fluorometry
fluorophotometry
Fluoroplex
fluorouracil (FU)
5-fluorouracil (5-FU)
Fluosol
Fluosol-DA 20%
FMEL (Friend murine erythroleukemia)
FMF (familial Mediterranean fever)
FNAB (fine-needle aspiration biopsy)
FOCMA (feline oncornavirus-associated cell membrane antigen)
folate
    deficiency anemia, f.
    level, f.
    storage, f.
Folex
folic acid
Folin's method

Folin and Wu's method
folinic acid
   rescue, f.
follicular dendritic cells
Fonio's solution
footprinting
foreign body
   giant cells, f.
foreign serum
Forestier's disease
forme fruste
formed elements
formyl-methionyl-leucyl-phenylalanine
Forssman
   antibody, F.
   antigen, F.
foscarnet
Foscavir
Fouchet's test
Fourneau 309
four-point assay
FPG (fasting plasma glucose)
fractionated
fractionation
fragellin
fragility
fragilocyte
fragilocytosis
fragment
fragmented cells
FRC (frozen red cells)
free
   base, f.
   erythrocyte coproporphyria, f. (FECP)
   erythrocyte coproporphyrin, f. (FECP)
   erythrocyte protoporphyrin, f. (FEPP)
   -floating clot, f.
   thyroxine, f. (FT4)
   thyroxine index, f. (FTI)
freebasing
Frei antigen
Frerich's theory
fresh frozen
   plasma, f. (FFP)

fresh frozen *(continued)*
   platelets, f.
Freund's
   complete adjuvant, F.
   incomplete adjuvant, F.
FRF (filter replacement fluid)
Friedlander's
   bacillus, F.
   pneumonia, F.
Friend
   leukemia cells, F. (FLC)
   murine erytholeukemia, F. (FMEL)
frozen
   plasma, f.
   red cells, f. (FRC)
fructosemia
FSF (fibrin-stabilizing factor)
FSP (fibrinogen OR fibrinolytic split products)
FTA (fluorescent treponemal antibody)
FTA-ABS (fluorescent treponemal antibody-absorption test for syphilis)
FT4 (free thyroxine)
FTI (free thyroxine index)
Ftorafur
FU (fluorouracil)
5-FU (5-fluorouracil)
FUdR (floxuridine OR fluorodeoxyuridine)
fugu toxin
full blood examination
FUM (5-FU and methotrexate)
fungal arthritis
fungemia
Fungilin
Fungizone
FUO (fever of unknown origin)
furazolidone
fusarial toxin
Fusarium
fusidic acid
Fusidin
Fv fragment

Additional entries

G

gadolinium diethylenetriamine-pentaacetate (Gd-DTPA)
gag gene
GAG (glycosaminoglycan)
Gaisbock disease
galactosemia
gallium
    nitrate, g.
    scan, g.
GaLV (gibbon ape lymphosarcoma virus)
Gamastan
Gambro Lundia Minor
Gamimune N
Gamiunen
gamma
    chain, g.
    counter, g.
    -Favre body, g.
    globulin, g.
    glutamyl transferase, g.
    HCD, g.
    heavy chain disease, g.
    interferon, g.
    peak. g.
    radiation, g.
Gammagee
gammaglobulinopathy
gammagram
gammagraphic
Gammar
gammopathy
Gamna-Gandy body
Gamulin Rh
ganciclovir sodium
Ganite
Gantanol
Gardner syndrome
Gardner-Rasheed sarcoma virus
gargle
gargling
gas gangrene toxin
gastritis
gastroenteritis
gastrointestinal
Gaucher disease
gay
    bar, g.
    -bashing, g.
    bowel infection, g.
    bowel syndrome, g.
    disease, g.
    lifestyle, g.
    lymph node syndrome, g. (GLNS)
    -related immunodeficiency diseases, g. (GRID)
G-banding
GBIA (Guthrie bacterial inhibition assay)
GCSA (gross cell surface antigen)
Gd-DTPA (gadolinium diethylenetriamine-pentaacetate)
gel
    filtration, g.
    plate, g.
gelatin sponge
Gelfilm
Gelfoam
gender
    assignment, g.
    change, g.
    dysphoria syndrome, g.
    role, g.
    -specific, g.
    testing, g.
gene
    allelic g.
    autosomal g.
    cell interaction g.(CI)
    CI g.
    cloned g.
    codominant g.
    complementary g.
    cumulative g.
    derepressed g.
    dominant g.
    env (envelope) g.
    gag g.

gene *(continued)*
  H g.
  histocompatibility g.
  holandric g.
  immune response g.(Ir)
  immune suppressor g.(Is)
  immunoglobulin g.
  inhibiting g.
  Ir g.
  Is g.
  leaky g.
  lethal g.
  major g.
  modifying g.
  mutant g.
  nonstructural g.
  operator g.
  pleiotropic g.
  pol g.
  recessive g.
  reciprocal g.
  regulator g.
  regulatory g.
  repressed g.
  repressor g.
  sex-conditioned g.
  sex-influenced g.
  sex-limited g.
  sex-linked g.
  sex-reversal g.
  silent g.
  structural g.
  sublethal g.
  supplementary g.
  suppressor g.
  syntenic g.
  tat g.
  transforming g.
  wild-type g.
  X-linked g.
  Y-linked g.
gene amplification
gene bank
gene cloning
gene code
gene complex
gene designing
gene flow
gene library
gene mapping
gene pool
gene repression
gene segment
gene sequencing
gene splicing
gene therapy
gene transcription
gene transfer
GeneAmp PCR test
genetic
  code, g.
  counseling, g.
  engineering, g.
  immunity, g.
  map, g.
  marker, g.
  masking tape, g.
  mutation, g.
  screening, g.
genetics
Gengou phenomenon
genital
  herpes, g.
  warts, g.
genitalia
genitaloid
genitoplasty
genome
  virus. g.
genomic
  library, g.
genotype
gentian violet
Gentran
  40, G.
  75, G.
German measles virus
Germanin
Germistan virus
germ-line
  DNA, g.
  theory, g.

GH3
ghost cell
giant
   cell, g.
   follicular lymphoma, g.
   platelets, g.
Gianturco-Roehm bird's nest vena cava filter
Giardia
   lamblia, G.
giardiasis
gibbon ape lymphosarcoma virus (GaLV)
Giemsa
   banding technique, G.
   stain, G.
Gignotti-Crosti syndrome
Gilbert phenomenon
gingivitis
gingivostomatitis
ginseng
Glanzmann's
   syndrome, G.
glass factor
glial cell
Glimepride
glitter cells
GLNS (gay lymph node syndrome)
globe cell anemia
globin
   gene, g.
globinometer
globoside
globulin
   AC g.
   accelerator g.
   alpha g.
   alpha 1 g.
   alpha 2 g.
   antidiphtheritic g.
   antihemophilic g. (AHG)
   antilymphocyte g. (ALG)
   antithymocyte g. (ATG)
   anti-human g. serum
   beta g.
   corticosteroid-binding g. (CBG)
   cortisol-binding g. (CBG)

globulin *(continued)*
   gamma g.
   hepatitis B immune g.
   immune g.
   immune human serum g.
   pertussis immune g.
   rabies immune g.
   Rho(D) immune g.
   testosterone-estradiol-binding g. (TEBG)
   tetanus immune g.
   thyroxine-binding g.
   vaccinia immune g. (VIG)
   varicella-zoster immune g. (VZIG)
   X, g.
globulin peak
globulose
glomerular basement membrane
glomerulonephritis
glomerulosclerosis
glossitis
GLQ223
glucagon
   stimulation test, g.
glucagonoma syndrome
Glucan
glucemia
glucocorticoid
Gluco-Ferrum
glucohemia
glucokinetic
glucokinin
Glucometer
glucopenia
glucose
   -6-phosphate dehydrogenase g. (G6PD)
   tolerance factor, g.
   tolerance test, g. (GTT)
glucosidase
glutamic
   -oxaloacetic transaminase, g. (GOT)
   -pyruvic transaminase, g. (GPT)
glutathione
   stability test, g.
glutathionemia

gluten
    fibrin, g.
    -sensitive enteropathy, g.
Glutose
glycan-phosphatidylinositol-specific phospholipase D (GPIPLD)
glycemia
glycemin
glycerin blood serum
glycerol
glycohemia
glycohemoglobin
glycolysis
glycolytic
glycophorin
glycoprotein
    41, g. (GP 41)
    120, g. (GP 120)
glycosaminoglycan (GAG)
glycosemia
glycosylated hemoglobin test
glycosylation inhibitor
glycyrrhizin
Gm
    allotype, G.
    antigen, G.
GM-CSF (granulocyte macrophage colony stimulating factor)
GMK (green monkey kidney)
GMP (guanosine monophosphate)
GMS (Gomori or Grocott methenamine silver)
gnotobiotic
goat's milk anemia
gold therapy
golden showers
Goldstein's hematemesis
Golgi apparatus
Gomori methenamine silver (GMS)
gonad
gonadal
    aplasia, g.
    dysfunction, g.
    dysgenesis, g.
    sex, g.
gonadectomize

gonadectomy
gonadial
gonadoblastoma
gonadoinhibitory
gonadokinetic
gonadopathy
gonadotropic
gonadotropin
gonococcal
    arthritis, g.
    gingivitis, g.
gonococcemia
gonococci (pl. of gonococcus)
gonococcus (pl. gonococci)
gonorrhea
Gonzales blood group
Good's syndrome
Goodpasture's syndrome
Gordon's elementary body
GOT (glutamic-oxaloacetic transaminase)
Gottron's papule
gout
gouty arthritis
Gower hemoglobin
Gowers' solution
GP
    24/26 antigen, G.
    41, G. (glycoprotein 41)
    120, G. (glycoprotein 120)
gp160 envelope
    envelope gene product, g.
    envelope protein, g.
GPIPLD (glycan-phosphatidylinositol-specific phospholipase D)
GPT (glutamic-pyruvic transaminase)
Graffi virus
graft-versus-host (GVH)
    disease, g. (GVHD)
    reaction, g.
Gram's stain
gram-negative
    bacilli arthritis, g.
gram-positive
Gram-Weigert stain
granular leukocyte
granuloblast

granulocyte
  colony-stimulating factor, g. (G-CSF)
  macrophage colony-stimulating factor, g. (GM-CSF)
  macrophage precursor, g.
  transfusion, g.
granulocytic
  hyperplasia, g.
  hypoplasia, g.
  leukemia, g.
  series, g.
granulocytopathy
granulocytopenia
granulocytopoiesis
granulocytopoietic
granulocytosis
granuloma
granulomatosis
granulomatous
granulopenia
granulosis
  virus, g.
grape cell
Graves' disease
gray (Gy)
gray platelet syndrome
green machine
Greenwald and Lewman's method
GRID (gay-related immunodeficiency diseases)
griseofulvin
Grocott methenamine silver (GMS)
Gross
  cell surface antigen, G. (GCSA)
  leukemia, G.
  leukemia virus, G.
  virus antigen, G.
ground itch anemia
group
  agglutination, g.
  agglutinin, g.
  precipitation, g.
  sex, g.
growth
  factor, g.
  hormone, g.

G-CSF (granulocyte-colony stimulating factor)
G-6-M
G6PD (glucose-6-phosphate dehydrogenase)
G691 protocol
G-suit
GTT (glucose tolerance test)
guaiac
guaiac'd
Guama virus
guanidinemia
guanosine
  cyclic phosphate, g.
  derivatives, g.
  diphosphate, g.
  monophosphate, g. (GMP)
  phosphate, g.
  triphosphate, g.
Guarieri's bodies
Guaroa virus
Gull's renal epistaxis
gum bleeding
Gunther's disease
Guthrie bacterial inhibition assay (GBIA)
GVH (graft-versus-host)
GVHD (graft-versus-host disease)
Gy (gray)
gynander
gynandria
gynandrism
gynandroid
gynandroid
gynandromorph
gynandromorphism
gynandromorphous
gynandry
gynecogen
gynecogenic
gynecoid
gynecomastia
gynecomastism
gynecoplastic
gynecoplasty

Additional entries

H

HA (hyaluronic acid)
HAA (hepatitis-associated antigen)
HaAg (hepatitis A antigen)
Haber's toxicologic principles
haem
haema
Haemate-P
Haemonetics Cell Saver
Haemophilus
   aegyptius, H.
   ducreyi, H.
   gallinarum, H.
Haemophilus B conjugate vaccine
Haemophilus influenzae (H flu)
Haemophilus pertussis vaccine (HPV)
Hafnia
   alvei, H.
Hagedorn and Jansen's method
Hageman factor (factor XII)
H agglutination
H agglutinin
HAHTG (horse antihuman thymus globulin)
hairpin loop
hairy
   cell, h.
   -cell leukemia, h.
   leukoplakia, h. (HLP)
   sore, h.
Haitian immigration
Halbrecht's syndrome
half-life
   plasma iron clearance, h.
half-time
Hall antidote
Ham test
Hamburger's phenomenon
Hammarsten's test
Hammerschlag's method
Hand-Schuller-Christian disease
Hanger's test
hanging-block culture
hanging-drop culture

Hanks balanced salt solution (HBSS)
Hansel's stain
Hansen's disease
Hantaan virus
H antigen
HAPA (hemagglutinating anti-penicillin antibody)
haploid
haplotype
hapten
   inhibition test, h.
haptoglobin
Hardy-Zuckerman 2 feline sarcoma virus
Harting bodies
Harvey sarcoma virus
Hashimoto's thyroiditis
Hassall's corpuscles
HAT medium
Hata phenomenon
Hataan virus
haupt-agglutinin
HAV (hepatitis A virus)
Hayem's solution
Hb Barts (Bart's hemoglobin)
HB (hepatitis B)
   HBAg (hepatitis B antigen)
   HBcAb (hepatitis B core antibody)
   HBcAg (hepatitis B core antigen)
   HBeAb (hepatitis B "e" antibody)
   HBeAg (hepatitis B "e" antigen)
   HBIg (hepatitis B immunoglobulin)
HBs (hepatitis B)
   HBsAb (hepatitis B surface antibody)
   HBsAg (hepatitis B surface antigen)
HBI (high serum-bound iron)
HBO2 (oxyhemoglobin)
HBSS (Hanks balanced salt solution)
HBV (hepatitis B virus)
HCD (heavy chain disease)
H cells
HCG (human chorionic gonadotropin)
H (heavy) chain
HCL (hairy-cell leukemia)

HCT (hematocrit)
HDCV (human diploid cell vaccine (HDCV)
HDL (high-density lipoprotein)
HDN (hemolytic disease of the newborn)
HDRV (human diploid cell rabies vaccine)
Heaf test
HEAT (human erythrocyte agglutination test)
heat exchanger
heat-killed (HK)
    Listeria monocytogenes, h. (HKLM)
heat-stable
    lactic dehydrogenase, h. (HLDH)
heavy
    chain, h. (H)
    ions, h.
    particle, h.
    polypeptide chains, h.
heelstick hematocrit
Heidenhain's iron hematoxylin stain
Heinz
    bodies, H.
    -body hemolytic anemia, H.
    granules, H.
Heinz-Ehrlich bodies
Hektoen phenomenon
HeLa cells
heliotrope erythema
HELLP (hemolysis, elevated liver enzymes, low platelets)
helmet cell
Helminthosporium
helper
    cells, h.
    -inducer cells, h.
    -suppressor cells, h.
    T-cells, h.
    virus, h.
hema
hemachrome
hemacytometer
hemacytozoon
hemad
hemadostenosis
hemadsorbent
hemadsorption
hemadynamometer
hemadynamometry
hemafacient
hemafecia
hemagglutinating
    antibody, h.
    anti-penicillin antibody, h. (HAPA)
    unit, h.
    virus of Japan, h.
hemagglutination
    inhibition, h. (HI)
    titer, h. (HT)
hemagglutinative
hemagglutinin
    inhibition, h.
hemal
hemalum
hemanalysis
hemangioblast
hemangioblastoma
hemangioblastomatosis
hemangioendothelioblastoma
hemangioendothelioma
hemangioendotheliosarcoma
hemangiofibroma
hemangioma
hemangiomatosis
hemangiopericyte
hemangiopericytoma (HPC)
hemangiosarcoma
hemapheic
hemaphein
hemapheresis
hemarthroses
hemarthrosis (hemarthroses)
hemartoma
hematal
hematapostema
hematein test
hematemesis
hematencephalon
Hematest
hematherapy
hematic

hematimeter
hematin
hematinemia
hematinic
    principle, h.
hematinometer
hematoblast
hematocele
hematochezia
hematochromatosis
hematocrit (HCT)
hematocryal
hematocrystallin
hematocyanin
hematocyte
hematocytoblast
hematocytolysis
hematocytometer
hematocytopenia
hematocytozoon
hematocyturia
hematodialysis
hematoencephalic
    barrier, h.
hematogen
hematogenesis
hematogenic
hematogenous
    pathways, h.
    spread, h.
hematoglobin
hematoglobinuria
hematoglobulin
hematogone
hematohistoblast
hematohyaloid
hematoid
hematoidin
    crystals, h.
hematologic
hematologist
hematology
hematolysis
hematolytic
hematoma
hematometer

hematometry
hematonic
hematopathology
hematopenia
hematophage
hematophagia
hematophagocyte
hematophagous
hematophilia
hematophobia
hematopiesis
hematoplastic
hematopneic
    index, h.
hematopoiesis
hematopoietic
    maturation alteration, h,
    maturation arrest, h.
    maturation stem cells, h.
    system, h.
hematopoietin
hematoporphyria
hematoporphyrin
    derivative, h. (HPD)
hematoporphyrinemia
hematoporphyrinism
hematorrhea
hematoscope
hematoscopy
hematose
hematosepsis
hematosis
hematospectrophotometer
hematospectroscope
hematospectroscopy
hematospherinemia
hematostatic
hematotherapy
hematotoxic
hematotoxicosis
hematotropic
hematoxic
hematoxylin
    body, h.
    -eosin stain, h. (H&E stain)
hematozemia

hematozoon
hematozymosis
hematuria
heme
   synthesis, h.
   synthetase, h.
hemic
hemin
hemizygosity
hemizygous
hemoagglutination
hemoagglutinin
hemobilinuria
hemoblast
hemoblastic
   leukemia, h.
hemoblastosis
hemocatheresis
hemocatheretic
Hemoccult test
hemochromatosis
hemochromatotic
   arthritis, h.
hemochrome
hemochromogen
hemochromometer
hemochromometry
hemochromoprotein
hemoclasia
hemoclasis
hemoclastic
hemocoagulin
hemoconcentration
hemoconia
hemoconiosis
hemocryoscopy
HemoCue photometer
hemoculture
hemocuprein
hemocyanin
hemocyte
hemocytoblast
hematocytoblastic
   leukemia, h.
hemocytoblastoma
hemocytocatheresis

hemocytogenesis
hemocytology
hemocytolysis
hemocytoma
hemocytometer
hemocytometry
hemocytophagia
hemocytopoiesis
hemocytotripsis
hemocytozoon
hemodiagnosis
Hemo-Dial dialysate additive
hemodialysis
hemodialyzer
hemodiapedesis
hemodiastase
hemodilution
hemodynamic
   crisis, h.
hemodynamometer
hemodynamometry
hemodystrophy
Hemofil
hemofilter
hemofiltration
hemoflagellate
hemofuscin
hemogenesis
hemogenic
hemoglobin (Hgb)
   A, h.
   A1c, h.
   A2, h.
   A/F, h.
   Bart's h.
   C, h.
   C-thalassemia, h.
   carbamate, h.
   Chesapeake, h.
   D, h.
   deoxygenated h.
   E, h.
   fast h.
   fetal h.
   glycosylated h.
   Gun Hill, h.

hemoglobin (Hgb) *(continued)*
  H, h.
  I, h.
  Lepore, h.
  M, h.
  mean corpuscular h.
  muscle h.
  nitric oxide h.
  oxidized h.
  oxygenated h.
  Rainier, h.
  S, h.
  Seattle, h.
  slow h.
  Yakima, h.
hemoglobin and hematocrit (H&H)
hemoglobin-binding capacity
hemoglobin cast
hemoglobin electrophoresis
hemoglobin hemochromogen
hemoglobin nadir
hemoglobinated
hemoglobinemetry
hemoglobinemia
hemoglobinocholia
hemoglobinolysis
hemoglobinometer
hemoglobinopathy
hemoglobinopepsia
hemoglobinophilic
hemoglobinorrhea
hemoglobinous
hemoglobinuria
hemogram
hemohistioblast
hemoid
hemokinesis
hemokinetic
hemokonia
hemokoniosis
hemolymph
    heteroagglutinin, h.
hemolysate
hemolysin
hemolysis
hemolytic

hemolytic *(continued)*
  anemia, h.
  complement assay, h.
  disease of the newborn, h. (HDN)
  icteroanemia, h.
  icterus, h.
  jaundice, h.
  plaque assay, h.
  -uremic syndrome, h.
hemolytopoiesis
hemolytopoietic
hemolyzable
hemolyzation
hemolyze
hemomanometer
hemometer
hemopathic
hemopathology
hemopathy
hemoperfusion
hemopexin
hemophage
hemophagocyte
hemophagocytosis
hemophil
hemophilia
  A, h.
  B, h.
  B Leyden, h.
  C, h.
  neonatorum, h.
hemophiliac
hemophilic
hemophilioid
hemophthisis
hemopiezometer
hemoplastic
hemopoiesic
hemopoiesis
hemopoietic
hemopoietin
hemopoietine
hemoprecipitin
hemoproctia
hemoprotein
hemopsonin

hemoptic
hemoptoic
hemoptysic
hemoptysis
Hemopump
hemorrhage
hemorrhagenic
hemorrhagic
    fever, h.
    measles, h.
    shock, h.
    thrombocythemia, h.
hemorrhagin
hemorrhagiparous
hemorrhea
hemosiderin
hemosiderinuria
hemosiderosis
hemospasia
hemostasia
hemostasis
hemostat
hemostatic
    plug, h.
Hemostix
hemostyptic
hemotherapy
hemotoxic
hemotoxin
hemozoin
hemozoon
hemuresis
Henle's fibrin
Henoch-Schonlein
    purpura, H.
    syndrome, H.
Henry test
hepadnovirus
heparin
    lock, h.
    sodium, h.
    sulfate proteoglycan anticoagulant, h.
heparinate
heparinemia
heparinize
hepatic

hepatitis
    A antigen, h. (HaAg)
    A virus, h. (HAV)
    B, h. (HB or HBs)
    B antigen. h. (HBAg)
    B core antibody. h. (HBcAb)
    B core antigen, h. (HBcAg)
    B immunoglobulin, h. (HBIg)
    B surface antibody, h. (HBsAb)
    B surface antigen, h. (HBsAg)
    B vaccine recombinant, h.
    B virus vaccine inactivated, h.
    B virus, h. (HBV)
    B "e" antibody, h. (HBeAb)
    B "e" antigen, h. (HBeAg)
hepatitis-associated antigen (HAA)
hepatobiliary
hepatocellular
hepatocyte
    -stimulating factor, h.
hepatomegaly
hepatosplenomegaly (HSM)
hepatotoxemia
hep-lock
Heptavax-B
heptoglobin
heptoglobinemia
herbal extract
herd immunity
hereditary
    erythroblastic multinuclearity, h.
    hemorrhagic telangiectasia, h.
    nonspherocytic hemolytic anemia, h.
        (HNSHA)
    persistence of fetal hemoglobin, h.
        (HPFH)
    plasmathromboplastin component, h.
    spherocytosis, h.
Hermansky-Pudlak syndrome
hermaphrodite
hermaphroditism
hermaphroditismus
heroin
heroinism
herpangina virus
Herp-Check

herpes
- anorectal h.
- corneae, h.
- digitalis, h.
- encephalitis, h.
- faciales, h.
- febrilis, h.
- genitalis, h.
- gestationis, h.
- gladiatorum, h.
- labialis, h.
- menstrualis, h.
- ocular h.
- ophthalmicus, h.
- pharyngeal h.
- progenitalis, h.
- simplex, h. (HS)
- traumatic h.
- virus simiae encephalomyelitis, h.
- wrestler's h.
- zoster, h.
- zoster auricularis, h.
- zoster ophthalmicus, h.
- zoster oticus, h.

herpes-like virus
herpes simplex virus (HSV)
- types I, II, h. (HSV I, II)

herpes-specific enzyme
herpes virus or herpesvirus
Herpesvirus (HV)
- hominis, H. (HVH)
- simiae, H.

herpes whitlow
herpes zoster virus (HZV)
herpetic
- gingivostomatitis, h.
- proctitis, h.
- sore throat, h.
- whitlow, h.

herpetiform
herpetiformis
herpetism
Herpex Liquifilm
Herrick's anemia
Herxheimer's reaction
Hespan

hetastarch
heteroagglutination
heteroagglutinin
heteroantibody
heteroantigen
heteroclitic
- antibody, h.

heterocliticity
heterocytotropic
- antibody, h.

heterodimer
heteroduplex
heterogeneic
- antigen, h.

heterogeneity
heterogenetic
- antibody, h.
- antigen, h.

heterogenous
- nuclear RNA, h. (hnRNA)

heterohemagglutination
heterohemagglutinin
heterohemolysin
heteroimmune
heteroimmunity
heteroinoculation
heterointoxication
heterokaryon
heterologous
- antigen, h.
- serum, h.
- vaccine, h.

heterolysin
heterolysis
heterolytic
heterophil
- antibody, h.
- antigen, h.

heterophile
- antibody, h.
- antigen, h.
- hemolysin, h.

heterophilic
- leukocyte, h.

heterosera
heteroserotherapy

heterosexual
heterosexuality
heterotopic
heterotoxin
heterotransplantation
heterotypic
   vaccine, h.
heterovaccine
heterozygote
heterozygous
   hemoglobinopathy, h.
   thalassemia, h.
heurteloup
Hexamita
hexavaccine
hexose monophosphate shunt
Heymann's nephritis
H flu (Haemophilus influenzae)
Hgb (hemoglobin)
H gene
HGG (human gamma globulin)
H&H (hemoglobin and hematocrit)
HHNC (hyperosmolar hyperglycemic
   nonketotic coma)
HHNK (hyperglycemic hyperosmolar
   nonketotic)
HHV-6 (human herpesvirus-6)
HI (hemagglutination inhibition)
   titer, H.
HIB (Haemophilus influenzae type B)
   HIB polysaccharide vaccine
Hickman catheter
Hicks-Pitney thromboplastin generation
   test
hidden determinant
high
   density lipoprotein, h. (HDL)
   molecular-weight neutrophil chemo-
      tactic factor, h.
   power field, h. (hpf)
   risk, h.
   -risk behavior, h.
   -risk group, h.
   -risk sex, h.
   serum-bound iron, h. (HBI)
   -voltage electrophoresis, h. (HVE)

high *(continued)*
   -zone tolerance, h.
hinge region
Hinton's test
hirudin
hirudiniasis
histaminase
histamine
   -fast, h.
   -fast achlorhydria, h.
   -releasing factor, h.
histaminemia
histaminergic
histanoxia
histidinemia
histioblast
histiocyte
histiocytic
   leukemia, h.
histiocytoma
histiocytosis
histochemical
histocompatibility
   antigens, h.
   complex, h.
   genes, h.
   locus, h.
histocompatible
histocyte
histocytic
   leukemia, h.
histocytosis
   X, h.
histodifferentiation
histofluorescence
histohematic connective tissue barrier
histohematogenous
histohypoxia
histoincompatibility
histoincompatible
histone
Histoplasma
   capsulatum, H.
   capsulatum polysaccharide antigen,
      H. (HPA)
histoplasmin

histoplasmoma
histoplasmosis
histothrombin
histotope
histotoxic hypoxia
HIV (human immunideficiency virus)
    HIV-1
    HIV-2
    HIV AC-1e vaccine
    HIV-AG (HIV antigen)
    HIV-antigen (HIV-Ag)
    HIV-associated
    HIV bands
    HIV dementia
    HIV-1 ELISA
    HIV embryopathy
    HIV encephalopathy
    HIV envelope protein
    HIV-induced
    HIV p24 antigen
    HIV-1 specific primer pair (SK38-39)
    HIV transmission
    HIV wasting syndrome
HIVAGEN test
HIVID
HIVIG (anti-HIV immune serum globulin)
HK (heat-killed)
HKLM (heat-killed Listeria monocytogenes)
HLA (human leukocyte antigen)
    HLA crossmatch
    HLA-A antigen (human leukocyte antigen A)
    HLA-B antigen (human leukocyte antigen B)
    HLA-B27
    HLA-C antigen (human leukocyte antigen C)
    HLA-D (human leukocyte antigen D)
    HLA-DR (human leukocyte antigen DR)
    HLA-DR 1 (human leukocyte antigen DR 1)
    HLA-DR 5 (human leukocyte antigen DR 5)

HLA (human leukocyte antigen) *(continued)*
    HLA-L (human leukocyte antigen L)
    HLA-linked disease
    HLA-typing
HLDH (heat-stable lactic dehydrogenase)
HLP (hairy leukoplakia)
HLT (human lymphocyte transformation)
HLTV (human T-lymphotropic retrovirus)
HLV (herpes-like virus)
HMA-CMV (human monoclonal antibody to cytomegalovirus)
hmRNA (heterogenous nuclear RNA)
HN2 (nitrogen mustard)
HNSHA (hereditary nonspherocytic hemolytic anemia)
Hodgkin's
    cells, H.
    disease, H.
    lymphoma, H.
    sarcoma, H.
HOE-BAY 964
Hoffmeister series
holandric genes
holistic
hollow fiber dialyzer
home O2 (home oxygen)
homing receptor
homocystinemia
homocystinuria
homodimer
homoerotic
homoeroticism
homoerotism
homogeneous
homograft
homologous
    antigen, h.
    series, h.
    serum, h.
    vaccine, h.
homology
    region, h.
    unit, h.
homophil
homophilic

homophobe
homophobia
homosexual
    panic, h.
    sexual intercourse, h.
homosexuality
Homo-Tet
homotransplantation
homozygous
    typing cell, h. (HTC)
hookworm anemia
Hoppe-Seyler test
horizontal transmission
Hormodendrum
hormonagogue
hormonal
    manipulation, h.
    therapy, h.
hormone
    assay, h.
    profile, h.
hormonogenesis
hormonogenic
hormonopoiesis
hormonopoietic
hormonoprivia
hormonosis
hormonotherapy
horn cell
horror autotoxicus
horse
    antihuman thymus globulin, h.
        (HAHTG)
    cell test, h.
    red blood cells, h. (HRBC)
hospice
host
    cell, h.
    defenses, h.
    mechanism, h.
    response, h.
    target site, h.
    vector system, h.
hot-cold hemolysin
Howell
    bodies, H.

Howell *(continued)*
    method, H.
Howell-Jolly bodies
HPA-23 (antimonium tungstate)
HPD (hematoporphyrin derivative)
hpf (high power field)
HPFH (hereditary persistence of fetal hemoglobin)
HPV (Haemophilus pertussis vaccine OR human papillomavirus)
HRBC (horse red blood cells)
HRIG (human rabies immune globulin)
HS (herpes simplex)
HSA (human serum albumin)
HSF (hydrazine-sensitive factor)
HSM (hepatosplenomegaly)
HSV (herpes simplex virus)
    I, II, H. (herpes simplex virus type I, II)
HT (hemagglutination titer)
HTACS (human thyroid adenylate cyclase stimulators)
HTC (homozygous typing cell)
HTLA (human thymus lymphocyte antigen)
HTLV (human T-cell leukemia OR lymphoma virus)
    -I, -II, -III, -IV, H.
    MA, H.- (HTLV membrane antigen)
    membrame antigen, H. (HTLV-MA)
    provirus, H.
Huber needle
HuIFN (human interferon)
human
    albumin, h.
    AML cell line, h.
    antihemophilic factor, h.
    chorionic gonadotropin, h. (HCG)
    diploid cell rabies vaccine, h. (HDRV)
    diploid cell vaccine, h. (HDCV)
    erythrocyte agglutination test, h. (HEAT)
    gamma globulin, h. (HGG)
    herpesvirus-6, h. (HHV-6)
    immunodeficiency virus, h. (HIV)
    interferon, h. (HuIFN)

human *(continued)*
    leukocyte antigen, h. (HLA)
    lymphocyte antigen, h. (HLA)
    lymphocyte transformation, h. (HLT)
    monoclonal antibody to cytomegalovirus, h. (HMA-CMV)
    papillomavirus, h. (HPV)
    rabies immune globulin, h. (HRIG)
    serum albumin, h. (HSA)
    skin peroxidase-labeled antibody immunofluorescence test, h.
    T-cell leukemia virus, h. (HTLV)
    T-cell lymphoma virus, h. (HTLV)
    T-cell lymphotropic virus type I, II, III, h. (HTLV I, II, III)
    thymus antiserum, h. (HUTHAS)
    thymus lymphyocyte antigen, h. (HTLA)
    thyroid adenylate cyclase stimulators, h. (HTACS)
    T-lymphocyte retrovirus, h. (HLTV)
humanized vaccine
Humatin
humoral
    antibody, h.
    antibody response, h.
    immune response, h.
    immunity, h.
Hunter's glossitis
Hunter-Sessions balloon
Hurthle cells
HUTHAS (human thymus antiserum)
Hu-Tet
HV (Herpesvirus)
HVE (high-voltage electrophoresis)
HVH (Herpesvirus hominis)
HVS (Herpesvirus simiae)
hyaline
    leukocyte, h.
    thrombus, h.
hyaluronic acid (HA)
H-Y antigen
hybrid
    antibody, h.
    cell, h.
hybridization

hybridoma
    antibody, h.
    cell, h.
hybridons
hydrazine-sensitive factor (HSF)
Hydrea
hydremia
hydroconion
hydrocortisone
Hydro-D
hydroperoxyeicosatraenoic acid
hydrops
    fetalis, h.
hydrothionammonemia
hydrothionemia
hydroxocobalamin
hydroxyapatite
hydroxychloroquine
hydroxyhaphthoquinone
5-hydroxytryptamine
hydroxyurea
hydroxyzine
Hykinone
Hymenolepis
    fraterna, H.
    nana, H.
hymenoptera
hypalbuminosis
hyper IgE
Hyperab
hyperalbuminemia
hyperaldosteronemia
hyperaldosteronism
hyperalonemia
hyperalphalipoproteinemia
hyperaminoacidemia
hyperammonemia
hyperamylasemia
hyperandrogenism
hyperargininemia
hyperazotemia
hyperbaric oxygen
    chamber, h.
hyperbeta-alaninemia
hyperbetalipoproteinemia
hyperbicarbonatemia

hyperbilirubinemia
hyperbradykininemia
hyperbradykininism
hypercalcemia
hypercalcitoninemia
hypercapnia
hypercarbia
hypercarotenemia
hypercellularity
hyperchloremia
hypercholesterolemia
hyperchromatic
   cell, h.
hyperchromemia
hyperchylomicronemia
hypercoagulability
hypercoagulable
hypercupremia
hypercythemia
hypercytochromia
hypercytosis
hyperemia
hypereosinophilia
hypereosinophilic
   syndrome, h.
hyperepinephrinemia
hypererythrocythemia
hyperestrogenemia
hyperferremia
hyperfibrinogenemia
Hyperforat
hyperfractionation
hypergammaglobulinemia
hypergastrinemia
hyperglobulinemia
hyperglucagonemia
hyperglycemia
hyperglycemic
   -glycogenolytic factor, h.
   hyperosmolar nonketotic, h. (HHNK)
hyperglyceridemia
hyperglycinemia
hyperguanidinemia
hyperhemoglobinemia
Hyper-Hep
hyperheparinemia

hypericin
hyperimmune
   globulin, h.
   plasma, h.
   serum, h.
hyperimmunity
hyperimmunization
hyperimmunoglobulinemia E
hyperinsulinemia
hyperiodemia
hyperkalemia
hyperketonemia
hyperkinemia
hyperlactacidemia
hyperlecithinemia
hyperleukocytosis
hyperlipemia
hyperlipidemia
hyperlipoproteinemia
hyperlithemia
hypermagnesemia
hypermetabolism
hypernatremia
hyperneocytosis
hypernitremia
hypernormocytosis
hyperorthocytosis
hyperosmolality
hyperosmolar
   hyperglycemic nonketotic coma, h. (HHNC)
hyperosmolarity
hyperoxemia
hyperoxia
hyperparathyroidism
hyperpepsinemia
hyperphenylalaninemia
hyperphosphatasemia
hyperphosphatemia
hyperphosphoremia
hyperpolypeptidemia
hyperpotassemia
hyperprebetalipoproteinemia
hyperproinsulinemia
hyperprolactinemia
hyperprolinemia

hyperproteinemia
hyperpyremia
hyperreninemia
hypersalemia
hypersarcosinemia
hypersegmented
hypersensitivity
hypersensitization
hyperserotonemia
hypersexuality
hypersplenic
    anemia, h.
hypersplenism
hypersusceptibility
hypertensinogen
Hyper-Tet
hyperthermia
hyperthrombinemia
hyperthyroxinemia
hypertriglyceridemia
Hypertussis
hyperuricemia
hypervaccination
hypervariable
hyperviscosity
hypervolemia
hypoalbuminemia
hypoaldosteronemia
hypoaldosteronism
hypoalonemia
hypoaminoacidemia
hypobetalipoproteinemia
hypobilirubinemia
hypocalcemia
hypocapnia
hypocarbia
hypocellular
hypocellularity
hypochloremia
hypocholesterolemia
hypochromemia
hypochromia
hypochromic
    erythrocyte, h.
    microcytic anemia, h.
hypochrosis

hypocitremia
hypocoagulability
hypocoagulable
hypocomplementemia
hypocupremia
hypocythemia
hypocytosis
hypodipsic hypernatremia
hypoelectrolytemia
hypoeosinophilia
hypoepinephrinemia
hypoestrogenemia
hypoferremia
hypoferric
    anemia, h.
hypoferrism
hypofibrinogenemia
hypogammaglobulinemia
hypoglucagonemia
hypoglycemia
hypoglycemic
    shock, h.
hypoglycemosis
hypogonadism
hypogranulocytosis
hypoinsulinemia
hypokalemia
hypolipemia
hypolipidemic
hypolipoproteinemia
hypoliposis
hypolymphemia
hypomagnesemia
hypomorph
hyponatremia
hyponeocytosis
hyponitremia
hypo-orthocytosis
hypo-osmolality
hypo-osmolarity
hypoparathyroidism
hypoperfusion
hypophosphatasia
hypophosphatemia
hypoplastic
    anemia, h.

hypoplastic *(continued)*
   bone marrow, h.
hypopotassemia
hypoproaccelerinemia
hypoproconvertinemia
hypoproteinemia
hypoprothrombinemia
hyporeninemia
hyposalemia
hyposegmentation
hyposensitization
hyposplenism
hypostasis
hypostatic
hypothermic
   perfusion, h.
hypothrombinemia
hypothyroid
hypothyroidism
hypothyrosis
hypotonic
   buffer, h.
   solution, h.
hypouremia
hypouricemia
hypovolemia
hypovolemic
   shock, h.
hypoxanthine
hypoxemia
hypoxia
hypoxic
   hypoxia, h.
hypoxidosis
HypRho-D
HZV (herpes zoster virus)

Additional entries

I

IA (immune adherence)
Ia (immune-associated)
    antigen, I.
IAHA (immune adherence agglutination assay)
iatrogenic
    anemia, i.
IBC (iron-binding capacity)
IBD (inflammatory bowel disease)
IBF (immunoglobulin-binding factor)
IBL (immunoblastic lymphadenopathy)
IC (immune complex)
ICC (immunocompetent cells)
ichoremia
ichorrhemia
icteroanemia
icterogenic
icterohematuria
icterohemoglobinuria
icterohemolytic
    icterohemolytic anemia
icterohepatitis
icterus
    gravis neonatorum, i.
    neonatorum, i.
    praecox, i.
IDA (iron-deficiency anemia)
Idamycin
idarubicin hydrochloride
IDAV (immunodeficiency-associated virus)
IDDM (insulin-dependent diabetes mellitus)
I deficiency factor
idioagglutinin
idioheteroagglutinin
idioheterolysin
idioisoagglutinin
idioisolysin
idiolysin
idiopathic
    hypochromic anemia, i.
    megakaryocytic aplasia, i.

idiopathic *(continued)*
    thrombocytopenic purpura, i. (ITP)
idiotope
idiotype
    -anti-idiotype network, i.
idiotypic
    antigen, i.
    variation, i.
idiovariation
idoxuridine (IDU)
IDS (immunity deficiency state)
IDTP (immunodeficient thrombocytopenic purpura)
IDU (injection drug user or 2'-deoxy-5-iodouridine or idoxuridine)
IEOP (immunoelectro-osmophoresis)
IEP (immunoelectrophoresis)
IF (immunofluorescence)
IFA (indirect fluorescent or immunofluorescent antibodyor immunofluorescent as
IFN (interferon)
    IFN-alfa-2a
    IFN-alfa-2b
    IFN-alfa-n1
    IFN-alfa-n3
    IFN-alpha
    IFN-An
    IFN-beta
    IFN-gamma
ifosfamide
IFRA (indirect fluorescent rabies antibody)
IFT (immunofluorescence test)
iG (immune globulin)
Ig (immunoglobulin)
    Ig3 antibody
    IgA (immunoglobulin A)
    IgD (immunoglobulin D)
    IgE receptor
    IgE (immunoglobulin E)
    IGF-I
    IgG (immunoglobulin G)

Ig (immunoglobulin) *(continued)*
    IgG2a antibody
    IgM (immunoglobulin M)
    IgM-RF antibody
    IgY (immunoglobulin Y)
Ig-synthesizing B-cell lymphoma
IH (infectious hepatitis)
IHA (indirect hemagglutination)
IHBTD (incompatible hemolytic blood transfusion disease)
IHSA (iodinated human serum albumin)
IIF (indirect immunofluorescent)
IIFA (indirect immunofluorescent antibody)
Ilheus virus
illicit drugs
IL (interleukin)
    IL-1 (interleukin-1)
    IL-2 (interleukin-2)
    IL-3 (interleukin-3)
    IL-4 (interleukin-4)
    IL-5 (interleukin-5)
    IL-6 (interleukin-6)
IM (infectious mononucleosis OR intramuscular)
IMAA (iodinated macroaggregated albumin)
IMED infusion pump
Imerslund syndrome
Imerslund-Graesbeck syndrome
Imferon
immature erythrocyte
immediate transfusion
immune
    adherence, i. (IA)
    adherence agglutination assay, i. (IAHA)
    agglutinin, i.
    antibody, i.
    -associated, i. (Ia)
    body, i.
    clearance, i.
    complex, i. (IC)
    conglutinin, i.
    cytolysis, i.
    deviation, i.

immune *(continued)*
    elimination, i.
    globulin, i.
    hemolysis, i.
    hemolytic anemia, i.
    interferon, i.
    lactoglobulins, i.
    markers, i.
    modulation, i.
    modulator, i.
    neutropenia, i.
    paralysis, i.
    reaction, i.
    response, i. (Ir)
    response gene, i.
    serum, i.
    serum globulin, i. (ISG)
    status, i.
    suppression, i.
    suppressor, i. (Is)
    suppressor gene, i.
    surveillance, i.
    system, i.
    system modulator, i. (IMREG-1)
    thrombocytopenic purpura, i. (ITP)
immunifacient
immunifaction
immunity
    acquired i.
    active i.
    adoptive i.
    antibacterial i.
    antitoxic i.
    antiviral i.
    artificial i.
    cell-mediated i.
    cellular i.
    community i.
    congenital i.
    cross i.
    familial i.
    genetic i.
    herd i.
    humoral i.
    infection i.
    inherent i.

immunity *(continued)*
   inherited i.
   innate i.
   intrauterine i.
   local i.
   maternal i.
   native i.
   natural i.
   nonspecific i.
   passive i.
   species i.
   species-specific i.
   T cell-mediated i.(TCMI)
   tissue i.
immunity deficiency state (IDS)
immunization
immunize
immunizing unit (IU)
immunoadhesin
immunoadjuvant
immunoadsorbent
immunoadsorption
immunoassay
immunobead
   -binding assay test, i.
immunobiology
immunoblast
immunoblastic
   lymphadenopathy, i. (IBL)
   sarcoma of B-cells, i.
   sarcoma of T-cells, i.
immunoblot test
immunoblotting
immunocatalysis
immunochemical
immunochemistry
immunochemotherapy
immunocompetence
immunocompetent
   cells, i. (ICC)
immunocomplex
immunocompromised
immunoconglutinin
immunoconjugate
immunocyte
immunocytoadherence
immunocytochemistry
immunocytometer
immunocytometry
immunodeficiency
   cellular i.
   combined i.
   common variable i.
   common variable unclassifiable i.
   human with short-limbed dwarfism i.
   human with thymoma i.
   primary i.
   severe combined i. (SCID)
   X-linked hyper-IgM i.
immunodeficiency-associated virus
   (IDAV)
immunodeficient
   thrombocytopenic purpura, i. (IDTP)
immunodepressed
   state, i.
immunodepression
immunodepressive
immunodermatology
immunodeviation
immunodiagnosis
immunodiffusion
immunodominance
immunodominant
immunoelectro-osmophoresis (IEOP)
immunoelectrophoresis (IEP)
   countercurrent i.
   counter-i.
   crossed i.
   Laurell technique i.
   radio-i.
   rocket i.
   two-dimensional i.
immunoelectrophoretic
immunoelectrotransfer
immunoferritin
immunofiltration
immunofixation
   electrophoresis, i.
   in agar, i. (Agar-IF)
immunofluorescence (IF)
   assay, i.
   microscopy, i.

immunofluorescence (IF) *(continued)*
    test, i. (IFT)
immunofluorescent
immunogen
immunogenetic genetics
immunogenetics
immunogenic
    determinant, i.
immunogenicity
immunoglobulin
    gamma A (IgA)
    gamma D (IgD)
    gamma E (IgE)
    gamma G (IgG)
    gamma M (IgM)
    gamma Y (IgY)
immunoglobulin alpha chain
immunoglobulin-binding factor (IBF)
immunoglobulin class
    switching, i.
immunoglobulin delta chain
immunoglobulin domain
immunoglobulin epsilon chain
immunoglobulin fold
immunoglobulin gamma chain
immunoglobulin gene rearrangement
immunoglobulin genes
immunoglobulin heavy chain
    gene, i.
immunoglobulin kappa chain
immunoglobulin lambda chain
immunoglobulin light chain
immunoglobulin mu chain
immunoglobulin subclass
immunoglobulin superfamily
immunoglobulinopathy
immunohematology
immunohistochemical
immunohistofluorescence
immunohistologic
immunoincompetent
immunologic
    competence, i.
    effect, i.
    enhancement, i.
    homeostasis, i.

immunologic *(continued)*
    imbalance, i.
    mechanism, i.
    memory, i.
    paralysis, i.
    surveillance, i.
    tolerance, i.
immunological
immunologically
    competent cell, i.
    privileged sites, i.
immunologist
immunology
immunomodulary
immunomodulation
immunomodulator
immunomodulatory
immunoparalysis
immunoparasitology
immunopathogenesis
immunopathologic
immunopathology
immunoperoxidase
immunophenotype
immunopotency
immunopotentiation
immunopotentiator
immunoprecipitation
immunoproliferative
    small intestinal disease, i. (IPSID)
immunoprophylaxis
immunoradioassay (IRA)
immunoradiometric
    assay, i. (IRMA)
immunoradiometry
immunoreactant
immunoreaction
immunoreactive (IR)
    glucagon, i. (IRG)
    human growth hormone, i. (IRhGH)
    insulin, i. (IRI)
    parathyroid hormone, i. (IPTH)
    substance P, i. (ISP)
immunoreactivity
immunoregulation
immunoregulatory

immunoresponsiveness
immunorestorative
immunoselection
immunosenescence
immunosorbent
immunostimulant
immunostimulation
immunosuppressant
immunosuppressed
immunosuppression
immunosuppressive
immunosurveillance
immunotherapy
immunotoxicology
immunotoxin
immunotransfusion
immunovar
ImmuRAID
IMP (inosine monophosphate)
impaired host defenses
IMREG-1 (immune system modulator)
imuthiol
in drag
in situ
    hybridization, i.
in vitro
    cell transformation test, i.
    clonogenic assay, i.
    correlations, i.
    kinetics, i.
in vivo
    adhesive platelet, i.
    correlations, i.
In (indium)
inactivated serum
inactivation
inactivator
inappropriate polycythemia
Inapsine
inbred strain
inclusion
    bodies, i.
    cell, i.
    criteria, i.
incoagulability
incoagulable

incompatible hemolytic blood transfusion disease (IHBTD)
incomplete antibody
increased capillary fragility
incubation
    period, i.
IND (investigational new drug)
indanedione
indicanemia
indicator cell
indifferent gonads
indirect
    agglutination, i.
    conjugate immunoperoxidase, i.
    Coombs' test, i.
    fluorescent antibody, i. (IFA)
    fluorescent rabies antibody, i. (IFRA)
    hemagglutination, i. (IHA)
    immunofluorescent, i. (IIF)
    immunofluorescent antibody, i. (IIFA)
    radioimmunoassay, i. (IRIA)
    transfusion, i.
indomethacin
indoxylemia
induced sputum test
inducer
    cell, i.
infantile genetic agranulocytosis
infection
    immunity, i.
infectiosity
infectious
    arthritis, a.
    hemolytic anemia, a.
    hepatitis, i. (IH)
    mononucleosis, i. (IM)
    wart virus, i.
infectiousness
infective
    thrombus, i.
inflammatory
    arthritis, i.
    bowel disease, i. (IBD)
    response, i.
influenza
    virus, i.

influenza *(continued)*
   virus vaccine, i.
influenzal
Infusaid
Infuse-A-Port
infusion pump
INH (isonicotine hydrazine)
inhalant
   antigens, i.
inhalation
inherent immunity
inheritance
inherited
   immunity, i.
inhibiting
   factor, i.
   gene, i.
inhibition
inhibitor
initiation factor
injection drug user (IDU)
innate immunity
inner bodies
innocent bystander
inocula (pl. of inoculum)
inoculable
inoculate
inoculation
inoculum (pl. inocula)
inoscopy
inosemia
inosine
   monophosphate, i. (IMP)
   pranobex, i.
inosinic acid
Inosiplex
INPX
In-111 scan
insect vector
insorption
insulin
   -dependent diabetes mellitus, i-
      (IDDM)
   -like growth factor, i.
insulinemia
Integra PBS Pageblot

integrase
integrated provirus
integrin family
inter-alpha-globulin
intercellular
interdigitating cells
interferon (IFN)
   -alpha, i.
   -alfa-n3, i. (Alferon N)
   -beta, i.
interfollicular cells
inter-heavy chain disulfide loop
interleukin
   interleukin-1 (IL-1)
   interleukin-2 (IL-2)
   interleukin-3 (IL-3)
   interleukin-4 (IL-4)
   interleukin-5 (IL-5)
   interleukin-6 (IL-6)
Intermedics Infusaid
intersex
intersexual
intersexuality
interstitial plasma cell pneumonia
intertropical anemia
intestinal flora
intrachain disulfide loop
intracellular
   toxin, i.
intracorpuscular
intracytoplasmic
   inclusion cells, i.
intraerythrocytic
intraglobular
intralesional
   Velban therapy, i.
intraleukocytic
intraperitoneal transfusion
intrathecal
intrauterine
   immunity, i.
   transfusion, i.
intravasation
intravascular
   consumption coagulopathy, i. (IVCC)
intravenation

intravenous (IV)
   drug abuser, i. (IVDA)
   drug administration, i.
   drug user, i. (IVDU)
   glucose tolerance test, i. (IVGTT)
Intra-Op autotransfusion system
intrinsic
   affinity, i.
   association constant, i.
   clotting reaction, i.
   factor, i.
   pathway, i.
intromission
Intron A
Intron C
Inv
   allotype, I.
   group antigen, I.
I invariant
invariant chain
inversion
invert
iodide peroxidase
iodinated
   human serum albumin, i. (IHSA)
   macroaggregated albumin, i. (IMAA)
iodination
iodophilia
iodoquinol
IPP (isopropyl pyrrolizine)
iproniazid
IPSID (immunoproliferative small intestinal disease)
iPTH (immunoreactive parathyroid hormone)
Ir (immune response)
   gene, I.
IRA (immunoradioassay)
Iretin
IRG (immunoreactive glucagon)
IRhGH (immunoreactive human growth hormone)
IRI (immunoreactive insulin)
IRIA (indirect radioimmunoassay)
iridescent virus
IRMA (immunoradiometric assay)

iron (Fe)
   assays, i.
   -binding capacity, i. (IBC)
   -binding protein, i.
   clearance, i.
   deficiency, i.
   deficiency anemia, i. (IDA)
   dextran, i.
   level, i.
   lung, i.
   overload, i.
   plasma, i.
   plasma clearance, i.
   poisoning, i.
   salts, i.
   storage disease, i.
   stores, i.
   studies, i.
   therapy, i.
   turnover, i.
   uptake, i.
irovirus
irradiation
irreversibly sickled cell (ISC)
Is (immune suppressor)
   gene, I.
ISC (irreversibly sickled cell)
Iscador
ischemia
ischemic
iscom
ISG (immune serum globulin)
island
isoagglutination
isoagglutinin
isoallotypic
   determinant, i.
isoamyl nitrite
isoanaphylaxis
isoantibody
isoantigen
isocomplement
isocytosis
isoelectric
   focusing, i.
   point, i.

isoenzyme
isogeneic
   antigens, i.
isograft
isohemagglutination
isohemagglutinin
isohemolysin
isohemolysis
isohydric
isohypercytosis
isohypocytosis
isoimmune
   hemolytic anemia, i.
isoimmunization
isolated heat perfusion
isolation
isoleucine
isoleukoagglutinin
isolysin
isolysis
isomerase
isoniazid
isonicotine hydrazine (INH)
isonormocytosis
isophil
   antibody, i.
isophile
   antigens, i.
isoprecipitin
Isoprinosine
isopropyl pyrrolizine (IPP)
isoproterenol
isoschizomer
isoserotherapy
isoserum
Isospora

Isospora *(continued)*
   belli, I.
isosporiasis
isostimulation
isotherapy
isotope
isotype
isotypic
   determinant, i.
   variation, i.
isovaleric
   acidemia, i.
isozyme
ISP (immunoreactive substance P)
Itaqui virus
ITP (idiopathic OR immune thrombocytopenic purpura)
itraconazole
IU (immunizing unit)
IV (intravenous)
IVAC volumetric infusion pump
IVAP (in vivo adhesive platelet)
IVCC (intravascular consumption coagulopathy)
IVDA (intravenous drug abuser)
IVDU (intravenous drug user)
IVGTT (intravenous glucose tolerance test)
IVIG (intravenous immune gammaglobulin)
Ivy
   bleeding time, I.
   method, I.
Ixodes
   dammini, I.

Additional entries

J

J (joining) chain
Jaksch's anemia
Japanese B encephalitis virus
Jarisch-Herxheimer reaction
Jarrow
jaundice
jaundiced
Jaworski bodies
JC
 papovavirus, J.
 virus antigen, J.
jennerian
jennerization
Jerne plaque
Jeryl Lynn mumps virus
jet
 injection, j.

jet *(continued)*
 nebulizer, j.
Jevity isotonic liquid nutrition
JH virus
Job syndrome
johnin
joining (J) chain
Jolly's bodies
Jones' criteria
Jones-Mote reaction
Josephs-Diamond-Blackfan syndrome
jugular bodies
Junin virus
juvenile
 cell, j.
 pernicious anemia, j.

Additional entries

K

K (killer)
Kabikinase
KAF (conglutinogen-activating factor)
kala-azar infection
kalemia
kaliemia
kaliopenia
kalium
kallidin
kallikrein
    -inhibiting unit, k. (KIU)
kallikreinogen
Kallman syndrome
kanamycin
K antigen
kaolin partial thromboplastin time (KPTT)
Kaplan-Meier survival curve
Kaposi's
    sarcoma, K. (KS)
    varicelliform eruption, K.
kappa
    granules, k.
    light chain, k.
Karnofsky
    performance scale, K.
    score, K.
Karpas T-cells
Karr method
Karroo syndrome
karyopyknotic index (KI)
karyotype
Kasabach-Merritt syndrome
kasai
Kashin-Beck disease
Katayama fever
Kauffmann-White scheme
Kawasaki disease
K cell
K-B cells
Ke (Kern)
Kell
    antibody, K.

Kell *(continued)*
    antigens, K.
    blood system, K.
Kell-Cellano blood group
Kellgren's disease
Kemerova virus
keratocyte
Kern marker
Kern's isotypic determinant
kernicterus
ketoacidemia
ketoconazole
ketone
    body, k.
    threshold, k.
ketonemia
ketonic
ketosis
Ketostix
ketotic
Kety-Schmidt method
keyhole-limpet hemocyanin (KLH)
KFAB (kidney-fixing antibody)
KI (karyopyknotic index)
Kidd
    antibody, K.
    blood group, K.
kidney-fixing antibody (KFAB)
killed
    HIV, k.
    measles virus vaccine, k. (KMV)
    vaccine, k.
    virus, k. (KV)
killer (K)
    cell, k.
    T-cell, k.
Kim-Ray Greenfield vena cava filter
kinetocyte
King-Armstrong unit
kinin
kininogen
Kinsey research data
Kinyoun stain

Kirsten sarcoma virus
Ki-67
Kitzmiller test
KIU (kallikrein-inhibiting unit)
Klacid
Klebsiella
    oxytoca, K.
    pneumoniae, K.
Kleihauer test
Kleinschmidt technique
Klenow's fragment
KLH (keyhole limpet hemocyanin)
Klinefelter syndrome
Klippel-Trenaunay syndrome
Km
    allotype, K.
    allotypic determinant, K.
    antigen, K.
KMV (killed measles virus vaccine)
Kobert's test
Koch's phenomenon
koha
Kolmer test

Konyne H T
Korean hemorrhagic fever
Korin fever
Kostmann syndrome
Kowa MDS
Kowarsky's test
KPTT (kaolin partial thromboplastin time)
Krebs' leukocyte index
KS (Kaposi's sarcoma)
    lesion, K.
Kumba virus
Kunkel syndrome
Kupffer's cell
KV (killed virus)
Kveim
    antigen, K.
    reaction, K.
K virus
KVO (keep vein open)
    -type I.V., K.
kwashiorkor
Kyasanur Forest disease virus

Additional entries

L

LA (latex agglutination OR lymphocyte-activating)
    cluster, L.
LAA (leukocyte ascorbic acid)
labeled antigen immunoperoxidase
labeling
    index, l.
labile
    factor, l.
lability
labrocyte
La Bross spot test
lactamase
lactated Ringer's solution
lactic
    acidosis, l.
    dehydrogenase, l. (LDH)
    dehydrogenase virus, l. (LDHV)
lacticemia
Lactobacillus
    casei factor, L.
    lactis Dorner factor, L.
lactoferrin
lactoglobulins
lactoside
lacunar cell
LAD (leukocyte adhesion deficiency)
Ladendorff's test
Laetrile
LAF (lymphocyte-activating factor)
LAI (leukocyte adherence inhibition)
LAIA (leukemia-associated inhibitory activity)
LAIT (latex agglutination-inhibition test)
LAK (lymphokine-activated killer) cells
laked blood
Laki-Lorand factor
laking
laky blood
Lallemand's
    bodies, L.
Lallemand-Trousseau bodies
lambda

lambda *(continued)*
    bacteriophage, l.
    chain, l.
    phage vectors, l.
lambliasis
lambliosis
laminarin sulfate
laminated thrombus
Lamprene
Lancefield
    classification, L.
    precipitation test, L.
lancet
Langat virus
Langerhans' cell
Langhans' giant cell
Lansing virus
LAP (leucine aminopeptidase OR leukocyte alkaline phosphatase)
large
    granular lymphocytes, l. (LGLs)
    undifferentiated cells, l. (LUCs)
Lariam
LAS (lymphadenopathy syndrome OR lymphadenopathy-associated syndrome)
Laserflow blood perfusion monitor
L-asparagine
Lassa fever virus
latency
latent
    iron-binding capacity, l. (LIBC)
    virus, l.
lateral thrombus
latex
    agglutination, l. (LA)
    agglutination-inhibition test, l. (LAIT)
    condom, l.
    dam, l.
    fixation test, l.
    flocculation test, l. (LFT)
    particle agglutination, l. (LPA)
    slide agglutination, l.

Latino virus
LATS (long-acting thyroid stimulator)
   -protector, L. (LATS-p)
lattice theory
laudanum
Laurell's rocket immunophoresis
LAV (lymphadenopathy-associated virus)
LAV/HTLV-III
lawn plate
lazy leukocyte syndrome
LCAT (lecithin-cholesterol
   acyltransferase)
L cell
L-chain (light chain)
LCL (lymphocytic leukemia OR lymphosarcoma)
LCM (lymphocytic choriomeningitis)
   virus, L.
LD (lymphocyte-defined)
   antigen, L.
LDH (lactate dehydrogenase)
LDHV (lactic dehydrogenase virus)
LDL (low-density lipoprotein)
LE (lupus erythematosus)
   cell, L.
   cell prep, L.
   factor, L.
lead poisoning
leaky gene
LEC-CAM (lectin cell adhesion molecules)
lecithin
   cholesterol acyltransferase, l.- (LCAT)
lecithinemia
lecithoprotein
lectin
LED (lupus erythematosus disseminatus)
Lederer's anemia
Lee-White clotting time
leeching
left shift
Legionella
   direct immunofluorescent antibody, L.
   pneumophila pneumonia, L.
legionellosis
legionnaires' disease

LeIF (leukocyte interferon)
Leiner's disease
Leishmania
leishmaniasis
leishmanicidal
Leishman
   chrome cells, L.
Leishman-Donovan bodies
Lennert's lymphoma
lentil
   agglutinin binding, l.
   lectin affinity chromatography, l.
Lentinan
lentivirus
Leon virus
Lepore
   trait, L.
   virus, L.
lepra
   cell, l.
   reaction, l.
lepromatous
   leprosy, l.
lepromin
leprosy
leptocyte
leptocytosis
leptospirosis
lesbian
lesbianism
lethal
   dose, l.
   gene, l.
lethality
letrazuril
Letterer-Siwe disease
Leu
   Leu-1
   Leu-M1 stain
   Leu-2
   Leu 2+ cells
   Leu +2a+ cells
   Leu-3
   Leu-7
   Leu-11
leucine aminopeptidase (LAP)

leucovorin
   calcium, l.
   rescue, l.
leucyl-tRNA synthetase
leukapheresis
leukemia
   acute nonlymphocytic l.
   acute promyelocytic l.
   adult T-cell l.
   aleukemic l.
   aleukocythemic l.
   basophilic l.
   blast cell l.
   blastic l.
   Burkitt-type acute lymphoblastic l.
   chronic granulocytic l.
   chronic myelocytic l.
   compound l.
   cutis, l.
   embryonal l.
   eosinophilic l.
   granulocytic l.
   Gross' l.
   hairy-cell l.
   hemoblastic l.
   hemocytoblastic l.
   histiocytic l.
   L1210 l.
   leukopenic l.
   lymphatic l.
   lymphoblastic l.
   lymphocytic l.
   lymphogenous l.
   lymphoid l.
   lymphoidocytic l.
   lymphosarcoma cell l.
   mast cell l.
   megakaryocytic l.
   micromyeloblastic l.
   monocytic l.
   myeloblastic l.
   myelocytic l.
   myelogenous l.
   myeloid granulocytic l.
   myelomonocytic l.
   Naegeli l.

leukemia *(continued)*
   non-B cell l.
   non-T cell l.
   nonlymphocytic l.
   null cell acute lymphocytic l.
   null cell lymphoblastic l.
   plasma cell l.
   plasmacytic l.
   pre-B acute lymphocytic l.
   pre-T acute lymphocytic l.
   prolymphocytic l.
   promyelocytic l.
   reticuloendothelial cell l.
   Rieder cell l.
   Schilling's l.
   smoldering l.
   splenomedullary l.
   splenomyelogenous l.
   stem cell l.
   subleukemic l.
   thrombocytic l.
   T-cell l.
   undifferentiated cell l.
leukemia-associated inhibitory activity (LAIA)
leukemia erythrocytosis
leukemia virus
leukemic
   cells, l.
   infiltration, l.
leukemid
leukemogen
leukemogenesis
leukemogenic
leukemoid
   reaction, l.
leukencephalitis
Leukeran
leukexosis
leukin
leukoagglutinin
leukoblast
leukoblastosis
leukocidin
leukocrit
leukocytal

leukocyte
  acidophilic l.
  adherence inhibition l.
  agranular l.
  basophilic l.
  endothelial
  eosinophilic l.
  granular l.
  heterophilic l.
  hyaline l.
  lymphoid l.
  mast l.
  motile l.
  neutrophilic l.
  nongranular l.
  nonmotile l.
  passenger l.
  polymorphonuclear l.
  polynuclear neutrophilic l.
  transitional l.
  Turk's irritation l.
leukocyte acid phosphatase stain
leukocyte adherence inhibition (LAI)
leukocyte adhesion deficiency (LAD)
leukocyte agglutinin
leukocyte alkaline phosphatase (LAP)
leukocyte alloantibodies
leukocyte antigens
leukocyte ascorbic acid (LAA)
leukocyte common antigen
leukocyte count nadir
leukocyte diapedesis
leukocyte differential count
leukocyte fraction
leukocyte G6PD deficiency
leukocyte inhibitory factor (LIF)
leukocyte interferon
leukocyte margination
leukocyte migration inhibition (LMI)
leukocyte movement disorder
leukocyte nuclear hyposegmentation
leukocyte-poor red blood cells
leukocyte transfusion
leukocythemia
leukocytic
  crystals, l.

leukocytic *(continued)*
  infiltrate, l.
  margination, l.
  marrow, l.
  maturation alteration, l.
  nuclear hypersegmentation, l.
  nuclear hyposegmentation, l.
  pyrogen, l.
  series, l.
leukocytoblast
leukocytoclastic
leukocytogenesis
leukocytoid
leukocytology
leukocytolysin
leukocytolysis
leukocytolytic
  serum, l.
leukocytoma
leukocytopenia
leukocytophagy
leukocytoplania
leukocytopoiesis
leukocytosis
  absolute l.
  agonal l.
  basophilic l.
  eosinophilic l.
  lymphocytic l.
  mononuclear l.
  neutrophilic l.
  pathologic l.
  physiologic l.
  pure l.
  relative l.
  terminal l.
  toxic l.
leukocytosis-promoting factor (LPF)
leukocytotactic
leukocytotaxis
leukocytotherapy
leukocytotoxic
leukocytotoxicity
leukocytotoxin
leukocytotropic
leukoderivative

leukodiagnosis
leukodystrophy
leukoedema
leukoedema
leukoencephalitis
leukoencephalopathy
leukoencephaly
leukoerythroblastic
 anemia, l.
leukoerythroblastosis
leukoerythrogenetic
leukogram
leukokeratosis
leukokinesis
leukokinetics
leukokinin
leukolymphosarcoma
leukolysin
leukolysis
leukolytic
leukomaine
leukomainemia
leukomainic
leukomatous
leukomonocyte
leukon
leukopathia
leukopedesis
leukopenia
leukopenic
 leukemia, l.
leukophagocytosis
leukophoresis
leukoplakia
leukopoiesis
leukopoietic
leukopoietin
leuko-poor red blood cells
leukoprecipitin
leukosarcoma
leukosarcomatosis
leukosis
leukotactic
leukotaxine
leukotaxis
leukothrombin

leukotoxic
leukotoxicity
leukotoxin
Leukotrap red cell storage system
leukotriene
leukovirus
leuprolide acetate
levamisole hydrochloride
levothyroxine
levulosemia
Levy, Rowntree, and Marriott method
Lewis
 antibodies, L.
 blood group, L.
 phenomenon, L.
Lewis and Benedict method
Lewissohn method
Lf unit
LFT (latex flocculation test
LGLs (large granular lymphocytes)
LGV (lymphogranuloma venereum)
Liacopoulos phenomenon
LIBC (latent iron-binding capacity)
Libman-Sacks endocarditis
Lichtheim plaques
LIF (leukocyte inhibiting factor)
LIFT (lymphocyte immunofluorescence
 test)
ligand
ligase
light
 chain, l. (L-chain)
 microscopy, l.
Lillie's hematoxylin
limit
 flocculation, l.
 flocculation, l. of
line of Zahn
linkage
 disequilibrium, l.
Linson electronic cell counter
Lioresal
LIP (lymphocytic interstitial pneumonitis)
lipacidemia
lipedema
lipemia

lipid
   -coated virus, l.
   cytosomes, l.
   histiocytosis, l.
   panel, l.
lipochromemia
lipohemarthrosis
lipohemia
Lipo-Hepin
lipoidemia
lipolysis
lipolytic
   hormone, l.
lipopolysaccharide
lipoproteinemia
lipoproteins
liposomal
   daunorubicin, l.
   gentamicin, l.
liposome
Liposyn II, III
lipovaccine
lipoxygenase
   pathway, l.
Lipschutz bodies
Liquaemin Sodium
liquid
   hybridization, l.
   nitrogen, l.
Listeria
   monocytogenes, L.
Listerine
listeriosis
lithemia
lithic acid
lithium carbonate
littoral cells
live
   vaccine, l.
   virus, l.
livedo
liver
   extract, l.
   function test, l.
   Lactobacillus casei factor, l.
LLD factor

L1210 leukemia
LM427 (ansamycin)
LMF (lymphocyte mitogenic factor)
LMI (leukocyte migration inhibition)
LN2 lymphocyte marker
loading
   dose, l.
   test, l.
local immunity
localized leukocyte mobilization
loci (pl. of locus)
locus (pl. loci)
   HLA, l. of
Loevit cell
Loffler's
   blood serum, L.
   eosinophilia, L.
L-ofloxacin
lomustine
Lone Star fever
long
   -acting thyroid stimulator, l. (LATS)
   terminal repeats, l. (LTR)
Lortorfer's
   bodies, L.
   corpuscles, L.
Lossen's rule
louping ill virus
low
   -density lipoprotein, l. (LDL)
   -power field, l. (lpf)
   zone tolerance, l.
LPA (latex particle agglutination)
LPF (leukocytosis- OR lymphocytosis-
   promoting factor)
lpf (low-power field)
L-phase variant
L-phenylalinine mustard
L (light) polypeptides
LSA2L2 chemotherapy
LSH (lymphocyte-stimulating hormone)
LTF (lymphocyte transforming factor)
LTR (long-terminal repeats)
Lucey-Driscoll syndrome
LUCs (large undifferentiated cells)
Lukes-Collins classification

Lunyo virus
lupoid
   hepatitis, l.
lupus
   band test, l.
   erythematosus, l. (LE)
   erythematosus disseminatus, l. (LED)
   nephritis, l.
Lutheran
   antibody, L.
   blood group, L.
Ly
   antigen, L.
   B antigen, L.
lycopenemia
Lyl B cell
Lyme
   arthritis, L.
   disease, L.
lymph
   cell, l.
   follicle, l.
   node, l.
   node biopsy, l.
   node permeability factor, l. (LNPF)
   node sampling, l.
   nodule, l.
   plasma, l.
lymphadenia
lymphadenitis
lymphadenopathy
   -associated syndrome, l. (LAS)
   -associated virus, l. (LAV)
   syndrome, l. (LAS)
lymphagogue
lymphapheresis
lymphatic
   blockade, l.
   leukemia, l.
   mesh, l.
lymphatolytic
   serum, l.
Lymphazurin
lymphnoditis
lymphoblast
lymphoblastic

lymphoblastic *(continued)*
   leukemia, l.
   lymphosarcoma, l.
lymphoblastoma
lymphoblastomatosis
lymphoblastosis
lymphocerastism
lymphocytapheresis
lymphocyte
   -activating factor, l. (LAF)
   blastogenic factor, l. (LBF)
   -defined, l. (LD)
   -depleted, l.
   immunofluorescent test, l. (LIFT)
   mitogenic factor, l. (LMF)
   proliferation test, l.
   recirculation, l.
   -stimulating hormone, l.
   subset, l.
   transformation, l.
   transforming factor, l. (LTF)
lymphocythemia
lymphocytic
   choriomeningitis, l. (LCM)
   inflammatory infiltrate, l.
   interstitial pneumonitis, l. (LIP)
   leukemia, l. (LCL)
   leukocytosis, l.
   lymphosarcoma, l. (LCL)
   series, l.
lymphocytoblast
lymphocytoma
lymphocytoma
lymphocytopenia
lymphocytopoiesis
lymphocytopoietic
lymphocytorrhexis
lymphocytosis
   -promoting factor, l. (LPF)
lymphocytotic
lymphocytotoxic
lymphocytotoxicity
lymphocytotoxin
lymphocytotropic
lymphogenous
   leukemia, l.

lymphogonia
lymphogranuloma
　inguinale, l.
　venereum, l. (LGV)
　venereum antigen, l.
lymphogranulomatosis
lymphohistiocytic
lymphohistioplasmacytic
lymphoid
　cells, l.
　depletion, l.
　hemoblast of Pappenheim, l.
　interstitial pneumonia, l.
　leukemia, l.
　leukocyte, l.
　stem cell, l.
lymphoidocyte
lymphoidocytic
　leukemia, l.
lymphokentric
lymphokine
　-activated killer (LAK) cells, l.
lympholysis
lympholytic
lymphoma
lymphomatoid
lymphomatosis
lymphomatous
lymphopenia
lymphopenic
　agammaglobulinemia, l.
lymphoplasmapheresis
lymphopoiesis
lymphopoietic
lymphoproliferative
lymphoprotease
lymphoreticular
　cells, l.

lymphoreticulosis
　inoculation, l. of
lymphorrhage
lymphosarcoma
　cell leukemia, l.
lymphotaxis
lymphotoxin
lymphotrophy
lymphotropic
lymphs (lymphocytes)
Lyon phenomen
lyophilization
lyophilized
lyotropic
　series, l.
Lypho-Med
lysemia
lysin
lysinogen
lysis
lysogen
lysogenic
　factor, l.
lysogenesis
lysogenicity
lysogeny
lysokinase
lysolecithin
lysozyme
lyssa
　bodies, l.
lysylbradykinin
Lyt antigen
lytes (electrolytes)
lytic
　lesion, l.
　virus, l.

Additional entries

M

M (macroglobulinemia)
   cell, M.
   component, M.
MAb (monoclonal antibody)
MAC (Mycobactium avium complex or membrane attack complex)
macaque
MacConkey agar
Machado test
Machado-Guerreiro test
Machupo virus
MACI (membrane attack complex inhibitor)
macroamylase
macroamylasemia
macrobiotics
macrocyte
macrocythemia
macrocytic
   anemia, m.
macrocytosis
Macrodex
macroflora
macroglobulin
macroglobulinemia (M)
macroleukoblast
macrolides
macrolymphocyte
macrolymphocytosis
macromethod of Wintrobe
macromolecular
macromolecule
macromonocyte
macromyeloblast
macronormoblast
macrophage
   activating factor, m. (MAF)
   agglutination factor, m. (MAggF)
   chemotactic factor, m. (MCF)
   cytotoxic factor, m.
   -derived growth factor, m.
   growth factor, m. (MGF)
   inhibitory factor, m. (MIF)

macrophage *(continued)*
   -mediated, m.
   migration inhibiting factor, m. (MMIF)
macrophagocyte
macropolycyte
macropromyelocyte
macroreticulocyte
macroscopic
   agglutination, m.
macrothrombocyte
macule
maculopathy
Madin-Darby canine kidney cells
maedivirus
MAF (macrophage activating factor)
MAggF (macrophage agglutination factor)
magnesemia
MAHA (microangiopathic hemolytic anemia)
MAI (Mycobacterium avium intracellulare)
maintenance drug
major
   agglutinin, m.
   gene, m.
   histocompatibility complex, m. (MHC)
Makonde virus
malabsorption syndrome
malaise
malakoplakia
malaria
malarial
   rosette, m.
   stippling, m.
male
   prostitute, m.
   pseudohermaphroditism, m.
Malin's syndrome
mammary tumor virus
m-AMSA

Mancini plates
mannitol
Mann-Whitney U test
mantle irradiation
Mantoux skin test
manual differential
MAO (monoamine oxidase)
MAOI (monoamine oxidase inhibitor)
MAP (megaloblastic anemia of pregnancy)
marantic
   thrombosis, m.
   thrombus, m.
marasmic
   thrombosis, m.
   thrombus, m.
Marburg
   agent. M.
   virus, M.
March disease
march hemoglobinuria
Marchand's cell
Marchiafava-Micheli disease
Marek's herpesvirus disease
marfanoid hypermobility syndrome
Marfan's syndrome
marginal granulocyte pool
margination
marijuana
Marinol
Marituba virus
marker
   chromosome, m.
marrow
   aspiration, m.
   biopsy, m.
   cell, m.
   platelets, m.
   transplantation, m.
masculation
masculinization
masculinize
masked virus
Mason Pfizer monkey virus (MPMV)
massive transfusion
mast

mast *(continued)*
   cell, m.
   cell leukemia, m.
   leukocyte, m.
MAST (military or medical antishock trousers)
   suit, MAST
   treatment, MAST
mastadenovirus
mastocytosis
masturbate
masturbation
Masugi nephritis
MAT (multiple agent therapy)
matagens
matched lymphocyte transfusion
maternal
   antibody, m.
   immunity, m.
maternohemotherapy
Matuhasi-Ogata phenomenon
maturation
   alteration, m.
   arrest, m.
   B cell, m.
Maurer's dots
maximum
   permitted dose, m. (MPD)
   tolerated dose, m. (MTD)
Mayaro virus
May-Hegglin anomaly
MBA (medical blood alcohol)
mBACOD
MBC (minimal bactericidal concentration)
MBP (myelin basic protein)
MC29 myelocytomatosis virus
McCoy's media
MCD (mean corpuscular diameter)
McDonough sarcoma virus
MCF (macrophage chemotactic factor)
Mcg isotypic determinant
MCH (mean corpuscular hemoglobin)
MCHC (mean corpuscular hemoglobin concentration)
M-component

McIndoe vaginal creation
McIndoe-Hayes construction of artificial vagina
McKrae herpes simplex virus
McLeod
    blood phenotype, M.
    phenotype, M.
MCT (mean corpuscular thickness)
MCTD (mixed connective tissue disease)
MCV (mean corpuscular volume)
MDP (muramyl dipeptide)
mean corpuscular
    diameter, m. (MCD)
    hemoglobin, m. (MCH)
    hemoglobin concentration, m. (MCHC)
    thickness, m. (MCT)
    volume, m. (MCV)
measles
    mumps, and rubella (MMR) virus vaccine, m.,
    mumps virus vaccine, m. and
    rubella virus vaccine, m. and
    virus vaccine, m.
mebendazole
meCCNU (semustine)
mechanocyte
mechlorethamine
MED (minimum effective dose)
mediate transfusion
mediated
mediator
mediator cell
medical blood alcohol (MBA)
Medisperse
Mediterranean
    anemia, M.
    lymphoma, M.
    variant (B-), M.
Medrate
Medrol
mefloquine
Megace
megakaryocyte
megakaryocytic
    hypoplasia, m.

megakaryocytic *(continued)*
    leukemia, m.
megakaryocytopoiesis
megakaryocytosis
megaloblast
    Sabin, m. of
megaloblastic
    anemia of pregnancy, m. (MAP)
    erythropoiesis, m.
megaloblastoid
megaloblastosis
megalocyte
megalocytic
    anemia, m.
megalocytosis
megalokaryocyte
megathrombocyte
megavolt (MeV)
megestrol acetate
Mektec 99
melanoma
melena
melenemesis
melenic
    stools, m.
MELI (met-enkephalin-like immunoreactivity)
melitemia
Meloxine
melphalan
membrane
    attack complex, m. (MAC)
    attack complex inhibitor, m. (MACI)
    filter, m.
    fluidity, m.
    immunoglobulin, m.
    Na-K exchange pump, m.
membranoproliferative glomerulonephritis (MPGN)
Memorial Sloan-Kettering protocol
memory cells
Mengo virus
meningococcal
    arthritis, m.
    polysaccharide vaccine, m.
meningococcemia

meningococci (pl. of meningococcus)
meningococcin
meningococcosis
meningococcus (pl. meningococci)
meningocyte
meningoencephalitis
meniscocyte
meniscocytosis
Mephyton
M/E ratio (myeloid/erythroid ratio)
6-mercaptopurine (6MP)
Meruvax
Mexican hat erythrocyte
mesalamine
mesna
Mesnex
mesolymphocyte
messenger
   molecule, m.
   RNA, m. (mRNA)
metabolic acidosis
metachromatic leukodystrophy
metachysis
metagglutinin
metaglobulin
metahemoglobin
metainfective
metaiodobenzylguanidine (MIBG)
metalloporphyrin
metamyelocyte
metamyelocyte
metaplasia
metaproterenol
metathrombin
metazoa
Metchnikoff's cellular immunity theory
met-enkephalin-like immunoreactivity
   (MELI)
meth (methamphetamine)
meth lab (where illicit drugs are made)
methadone
methalbumin
methamphetamine
methaqualone
methemalbumin
methemalbuminemia

metheme
methemoglobin
   reductase, m. (NADPH)
   reduction test, m.
methemoglobinemia
methemoglobinuria
methenamine silver staining
methionine-enkephalin
methisazone
methotrexate (MTX)
methyl violet
methylene blue
methylprednisolone
methyltestosterone
metmyoglobin
metronidazole
metroplasty
MeV (megavolt)
Mexate
mexiletine
Meyer-Betz disease
MFD (minimum fatal dose)
MG (myasthenia gravis)
   agglutinin, M.
MGF (macrophage growth factor)
MHA-TP (microhemagglutination assay-
   Treponema pallidum)
MHC (major histocompatibility complex)
MHD (minimum hemolytic dose)
MIBG (metaiodobenzylguanidine)
miconazole
microaggregate
microangiopathic
   hemolytic anemia, m. (MAHA)
microangiopathy
microbe
microbial
microbicidal
microbiological
   assay, m.
microcytase
microcyte
microcythemia
microcytic
   anemia, m.
microcytosis

microcytotoxicity
microdrepanocytic
 anemia, m.
microdrepanocytosis
microdroplet
microelectrophoresis
microerythrocyte
microflora
microfluidity
MicroGeneSep
microglobulin
microhemagglutination assay-Treponema
 pallidum (MHA-TP)
microhematocrit
microimmunofluorescent test
microleukoblast
microlymphoidocyte
micromyeloblast
micromyeloblastic
 leukemia, m.
micromyelolymphocyte
micronormoblast
microorganism
microphage
microphagocyte
microrefractometer
microscopic
 agglutination, m.
 indices, m.
microscopy
microspherocyte
microspherocytosis
microsporidiosis
Microsulfon
microtiter
microtonometer
microtransfusion
microvasculopathy
MID (minimum infective dose)
Middlebrook's
 agar, M.
 broth, M.
Middlebrook-Dubos hemagglutination
 test
MIF (microphage inhibitory factor)
migration inhibitory factor

migratory cells
Mikulicz's syndrome
milk
 anemia, m.
 factor, m.
milker's node virus
Millipore filter
miloxantrone Hl
miner's anemia
minimal bactericidal concentration
 (MBC)
minimum
 effective dose, m. (MED)
 hemolytic dose, m. (MHD)
 infective dose, m. (MID)
 reacting dose, m. (MRD)
Minitec
minocycline
minor agglutinin
Minot-Murphy diet
mioplasmia
mismatch
missense mutation
mistaken gender identity
mistletoe extract
mithramycin
mitochondrial antibody
mitogen
mitogenic
 factor, m.
mitogenicity
mitomycin
mitosis
mitotic
mitoxantrone
Mitsuda antigen
mixed
 connective tissue disease, m. (MCTD)
 lymphocyte culture, m. (MLC)
 lymphocyte reaction, m. (MLR)
 thrombus, m.
 vaccine, m.
MKV (killed-measles vaccine)
MLC (mixed lymphocyte culture)
MLR (mixed lymphocyte reaction)
MLV (mouse leukemia virus)

MM virus
MM-1
MMIF (macrophage migration inhibiting factor)
MMR (measles, mumps, and rubella) virus vaccine, M.
MMTV (mouse mammary tumor virus)
MNSs blood group
MO2 Leu-M21 antibodies
MoAB (monoclonal antibody)
Mobin-Uddin filter
modifying gene
moiety
molality
molarity
molecular
  cloning, m.
  disease, m.
  genetics, m.
  hybridization probe, m.
  lesion, m.
  mimicry, m.
  weight, m.
molecule
Mol-Iron
molluscum contagious virus
Moloney
  test, M.
  leukemogenic virus, M.
  sarcoma virus, M. (MSV)
  test, M.
Molulsky dye reduction test
Monilia
monilial
  esophagitis, m.
moniliasis
moniliid
moniliosis
Monistat
monkey B virus
monkeypox virus
mono (infectious mononucleosis)
monoamine oxidase (MAO)
  inhibitor, m. (MAOI)
monoarticular arthritis
monoblast

monoblastic
  leukemia, m.
monoblastoma
Monoclate
monoclonal
  antibody, m. (MAb)
  antineurofilament antibody, m.
  band, m.
  gammopathy, m.
  immunoglobulin, m.
  spike,
monocyte
  -macrophage, m.
monocytic
  leukemia, m.
  marrow, m.
  series, m.
monocytoid
monocytopenia
monocytopoiesis
monocytosis
Mono-Diff test
monogamous bivalency
monogen
monohistiocytic
Monojector
monokine
monolaurin
monolayer
monomer
mononeuritis
  multiplex, m.
mononuclear
  cell, m.
  leukocytosis, m.
  phagocyte system, m. (MPS)
mononucleate
mononucleosis
  -like, m.
mononucleotide
monophyletic theory
Monos (monocytes)
Monospot test
monotherapy
monovalent
  oral poliovirus vaccine, m. (MOPV)

monovalent *(continued)*
  serum, m.
Mooser cell
8-MOP
MOPV (monovalent oral poliovirus vaccine)
Moranyl
Moraxella
  bovis, M.
  liquefaciens, M.
morbillivirus
Morgagni's column
morphea
morphine sulfate (MS)
morphinism
morphological sex
morphology
morrhuate sodium
morular cell
mosaicism
Mosse's syndrome
Mossuril virus
mother cell
motile serum
motility
Mott
  bodies, M.
  cell, M.
mountain anemia
mouse
  erythroleukemia, m.
  germ line DNA, m.
  leukemia virus, m. (MLV)
  mammary tumor factor, m.
  mammary tumor virus, m.
  myeloma cells, m.
  specific lymphocyte antigen, m. (MSLA)
  unit, m. (MU)
mouth cells
mouthrinse
mouthwash
moving boundary electrophoresis
6-MP (6-mercaptopurine)
MPD (maximum permitted dose)
MPGN (membranoproliferative glomerulonephritis)
MPMV (Mason Pfizer monkey virus)
MPO (myeloperoxidase)
M-protein
MPS (mononuclear phagocyte system)
MRD (minimum reacting dose)
mRNA (messenger RNA)
  interleukin 2, m.
  transcription, m.
  translation, m.
MS (morphine sulfate)
MS-Contin
MS-1 hepatitis
MS-2 hepatitis
MSL-109
MSLA (mouse-specific lymphocyte antigen)
MSOF (multiple systems organ failure)
MSV (Moloney sarcoma virus)
MTB (Mycobacterium tuberculosis)
MTD (maximum tolerated dose)
MTP-PE
MTX (methotrexate)
mu
  chain, m.
  HCD, m.
  receptors, m.
MU (mouse unit)
mucicarmine staining
mucinemia
mucocutaneous
  herpes, m.
mucopolypeptide
mucopolysaccharide
mucosa
mucosal
  absorption, m.
  transudate, m.
mucositis
mucosocutaneous
mucous
  colitis, m.
  enteritis, m.
  membrane, m.
mucus

Muercke's lines
Muller's dust bodies
multifactorial
multimer
multinucleated
multiple
   agent therapy, m. (MAT)
   -drug resistance, m.
   -drug therapy, m.
   myeloma, m.
   systems organ failure, m. (MSOF)
multivalent
multivesicular
mumps
   virus, m.
   virus vaccine, m.
Mumpsvax
mural thrombus
muramidase
muramyl dipeptide (MDP)
murine
   erythroleukemia, m.
   leukemia virus, m.
   sarcoma virus, m.
   T cell phenotype, m.
murivirus
Muromonab-CD3
Murray Valley encephalitis virus
Murri disease
muscle
   hemoglobin, m.
   plasma, m.
Mustargen
mutagenesis
mutagenic
mutant
   gene, m.
mutate
mutation
mutogenicity
mutual masturbation
Myambutol
myasthenia gravis (MG)
Mycelex
mycethemia
mycoagglutinin

mycobacteria
mycobacterial
   arthritis, m.
mycobacteriosis
Mycobacterium
   avium complex, M. (MAC)
   avium intracellulare, M. (MAI)
   kansasii, M.
   tuberculosis, M. (MTB)
mycohemia
Mycoplasma
   incognitus, M.
mycoplasmal
Mycosel agar
mycosis
   fungoides, m.
Mycostatin
mycotic
   stomatitis, m.
Mycotoruloides
mycotoxinization
myelemia
myelin basic protein (MBP)
myeloblast
myeloblastemia
myeloblastic
   leukemia, m.
myeloblastosis
myelocyte
myelocythemia
myelocytic
   leukemia, m.
   series, m.
myelocytomatosis
myelocytosis
myelodysplasia
myelodysplastic
   syndrome, m.
myelofibrosis
   -osteosclerosis syndrome, m.
myelogenous
   leukemia, m.
myeloid
   cell, m.
   -erythroblast ratio, m.
   -erythroid ratio, m. (M/E ratio)

myeloid *(continued)*
 granulocytic leukemia, m.
 leukemia, m.
 metaplasia, m.
 series, m.
myeloma
 cell, m.
 protein, m.
myelomatosis
myelomonocytic
 leukemia, m.
myeloneuropathy
myelopathic
 anemia, m.
 polycythemia, m.
myelopathy
myeloperoxidase (MPO)
myelophthisic
 anemia, m.
myeloplast
myelopoiesis
myeloproliferative
myelosis
myelosuppressed
myelosuppression
myelosuppressive
myelotoxic
myelotoxicity
myelotoxin
Myleran
myocyte
myoglobin
myoglobinuria
myoglobulin
myoglobulinuria
myohemoglobin
myosin
 ATPase, m.
 fibrin, m.
myxemia
myxovirus

Additional entries

N

NA (neutralizing antibody)
NAC (N-acetyl-L-cysteine)
NAD (nicotinamide adenine dinucleotide)
NADH (reduced form of NAD)
    dehydrogenase, N.
    diaphorase, N.
    methemoglobin reductase, N.
    oxidase, N.
nadir
NADP (nicotinamide-adenine dinucleotide phosphate)
NADPH (reduced form of NADP)
    ferrihemoprotein reductase, N.
    methemoglobin reductase, N.
    oxidase, N.
Naegeli's leukemia
NAG vibrios
Naganol
Nageotte's cells
Na-K exchange pump
Nakiwogo virus
NALL (null cell acute lymphocytic leukemia)
naltrexone
NANB (non-A, non-B) hepatitis
nanogram
nanoparticle
naphthylesterase-positive leukemic cells
Naphuride
naproxen
nasal insulin
National Institute of Allergy and Infectious Disease (NIAID)
native immunity
natural
    antibody, n.
    cytotoxic (NC) cells, n.
    immunity, n.
    selection theory, n.
natural killer (NK) cell
Nazlin
NBS (normal blood serum)
NBT (nitroblue tetrazolium)

N-butyl-deoxynojirimycin
NC (natural cytotoxic) cells
NCF (neutrophil chemotactic factor)
NDA (new drug application)
NDK
nebulization
nebulizer
NebuPent
necrotoxin
needle tracks
needlestick
nef (negative factor)
Negri bodies
Neill-Mooser
    body, N.
    reaction. N.
Neisser's granules
Neisser-Wechsberg leukocidin
Neisseria
    gonorrhoeae, N.
    meningitides, N.
neisseria mucosa
neisserial
neoadjuvant chemotherapy
neoantigen
Neo-Betalin 12
neocytosis
neonatal
    jaundice, n.
    lupus, n.
neoplasia
neoplasm
neoplastic
neopterin
Neosar
nephelometric
    immunoassay, n.
    inhibition assay, n.
nephelometry
nephritic
    factor, n.
nephritis
nephronophthisis

nephropathy
nephropoietin
nephrosclerosis
nephrotic syndrome
nephrotoxic
    antibody, n.
    serum, n.
nephrotoxicity
nephrotoxin
Netromycin
network theory
Neufeld's reaction
Neumann's cells
neuraminidase
neurohormone
neuroimmunology
Neuroleukin
neuropathic
    arthritis, n.
neuropathy
neuroradiological
neurosyphilis
neurotropic
    virus, n.
neurotropin
neurovaccine
neutralization
neutralizing antibody (NA)
neutrocytopenia
neutropenia
neutrophil
    chemotactic factor, n. (NCF)
    lobe count, n.
neutrophilia
neutrophilic
    cell, n.
    leukemia, n.
    leukocytosis, n.
    lymphycytosis, n.
    series, n.
New tuberculin
New Zealand black mouse (NZBM)
newborn pneumonitis virus
Newcastle disease virus
Nezelof syndrome
NHL (non-Hodgkin's lymphoma)

NHS (normal horse or human serum)
Niagestin
NIAID (National Institute of Allergy and Infectious Disease)
nick translation
nicotinamide-adenine
    dinucleotide, n. (NAD)
    dinucleotide phosphate, n. (NADP)
NIDDM (noninsulin-dependent diabetes mellitus)
Niemann-Pick disease
night sweats
Nikiforoff method
nimodipine
nine-mile fever
Nippe's test
nitavirus
nitric oxide hemoglobin
nitroblue tetrazolium (NBT)
nitrofurantoin
nitrogen mustard (HN2)
nitrosourea
Nizoral
NK (natural killer)
    cell, N.
N-linked glycosylation sites
N-Multistix
Nocardia
    asteroides, N.
nocardiosis
Noguchi's test
nonadherent cell
nonagglutinating
    vibrios, n.
nonalpha chain
non-A, non-B hepatitis (NANB hepatitis)
non-B-cell leukemia
non-B hepatitis
non-Burkitt's lymphoma
noncleaved
nonfilamented neutrophils
nongonococcal bacterial arthritis
non-Hodgkin's lymphoma
noninsulin-dependent diabetes mellitus (NIDDM)
nonlymphocytic leukemia

nonneoplastic
nonnucleated
nononcogenic virus
nonoxynol-9
nonphotochromogen
nonprecipitation antibody
nonprotein nitrogen (NPN)
nonradioisotopic
nonreactivity
nonsecretor
nonself
nonsense codons
nonsteroidal anti-inflammatory drug (NSAID)
nonspecific immunity
nonstructural gene
non-T-cell leukemia
nontreponemal spirochetes
nontypable
normal
    blood serum, n. (NBS)
    horse serum, n. (NHS)
    human plasma, n.
    human serum, n. (NHS)
    lymphocyte transfer test, n.
    rabbit serum, n.
normoblast
normoblastosis
normocalcemia
normocapnia
normocholesterolemia
normochromasia
normochromia
normochromic
    erythrocyte, n.
normocyte
normocytic
    normochromic anemia, n.
Normocytin
normocytosis
normoerythrocyte
normoglycemia
normokalemia
normo-orthocytosis
normoskeocytosis
normouricemia

normovolemia
Norport pump
Norris' corpuscles
Northern
    blot test, N.
    blotting, N.
Norwalk
    agent, N.
    virus, N.
nosocomial
    anemia, n.
nosohemia
nosotherapy
nosotoxic
notifiable disease
not-self
Novantrone
NPDL (nodular, poorly differentiated lymphocytes)
NPN (nonprotein nitrogen)
NRBC (nucleated red blood cell)
nRNA (nuclear RNA)
NSAIDs (nonsteroidal anti-inflammatory drugs)
Ntaya virus
N-terminal constant region
nuclear
    antigen, n.
    envelope, n.
    medicine, n.
    particles, n.
    RNA, n. (nRNA)
nuclease
nucleated
    erythrocyte, n.
    red blood cell, n. (NRBC)
    red cells, n.
nucleic acid
nuclein
    bases, n.
nucleocapsid
nucleoid
nucleoside
    analogue, n.
    phosphorylase, n.
nucleotidase

nucleotide
nucleotidyl
nucleotoxin
nude mice
null cell
    acute lymphocytic leukemia, n. (NALL)
    lymphoblastic leukemia, n.

null cell *(continued)*
    type non-Hodgkin's lymphoma, n.
nurse cell
nutritional anemia
nystatin
    pastilles, n.
NZB mouse (New Zealand black mouse)

Additional entries

O

O agglutination
O agglutinin
O antigen
O antistreptolysin
O2 sat (oxygen saturation)
OAF (osteoclast-activating factor)
Oakley-Fulthorpe technique
oat cell
Obecalp
obligate anaerobe
obscuration
obstructive thrombus
occluding thrombus
occlusive thrombus
occult blood
ochronosis
O-core polysaccharide
octreotide
ocular herpes
OD (overdose)
OD'd (overdosed)
odynophagia
ofloxacin
ohne Hauch
OI (opportunistic infection OR osteogenesis imperfecta)
OID (optimal immunomodulating dose)
OK 10 virus
OK-432 (picibanil)
OKT3, 4, 4A, 5, 8 antigen
old thrombus
Old tuberculin (OT)
oligemia
oligochromemia
oligoclonal
oligodeoxynecleotides
oligohemia
oligoleukocythemia
oligosaccharide
Oliver-Rosalki method
olsalazine
Ommaya reservoir
Omsk hemorrhagic fever virus
onanism
oncofetal
   antigen, o.
   proteins, o.
oncogene
   activation, o.
   peptide growth factor, o.
oncogenesis
oncogenetic
oncogenic virus
oncogenicity
oncotropic
Oncovin
oncovirus
One-Alpha
one-dimensional
   double electroimmunodiffusion, o.
   single electroimmunodiffusion, o.
One-Touch blood glucose meter
O'nyong-nyong virus
open label
   protocol, o.
   study, o.
   treatment, o.
O&P (ova and parasites)
open reading frame (ORF)
operator
   gene, o.
   locus, o.
opportunist
   infection, o. (OI)
   organism, o.
opsinogen
opsonic
opsonin
opsonization
opsonize
opsonizing antibodies
opsonocytophagic
opsonometry
opsonophilia
opsonotherapy
optical density

Opti-fluor
optimal immunomodulating dose (OID)
OPV (poliovirus vaccine live oral)
oral
    candidiasis, o.
    copulation, o.
    eroticism, o.
    intercourse, o.
    poliovaccine, o.
    poliovirus vaccine, o.
    sex, o.
    thrush, o.
    thrust, o.
    warts, o.
orality
OraQuick test
OraSure test
orbivirus
ordure
orf virus
ORF (open reading frame)
organ
    perfusion system, o.
    -specific antigen, o.
    transplant, o.
organelles
organized thrombus
organotropism
Oriboca virus
original antigenic sin
Orimune
ornithosis virus
orogenital
Oropouche virus
orotherapy
Oroya fever
orphan
    drug, o.
    virus, o.
orrhology
orrhoreaction
orrhotherapy
orthochromatic
    erythroblasts, o.
    erythrocytes, o.
orthoglycemic

Ortho-mune antibody
orthomyxovirus
orthopoxvirus
orthotopic
Osgood-Schlatter disease
Osmitrol
osmolal clearance
osmolality
osmolar
osmolarity
osmole
osmolute
osmometer
osmometry
osmosis
osmotic
    fragility, o.
    minipump, o.
O-specific polysaccharide
osteoclast-activating factor (OAF)
osteogenesis
    imperfecta, o. (OI)
osteomalacia
osteomyelitis
osteonecrosis
osteoporosis
osteoporotic
osteosclerosis
osteosclerotic
    anemia, o.
OT (Old Tuberculin)
Ouchterony
    double diffusion technique, O.
    immunodiffusion, O.
Oudin immunodiffusion
outbreeding
ova and parasites (O&P)
Ovaban
ovalocytosis
overdose (OD)
overdosed (OD'd)
ox
    cell hemolysin test, o.
    red blood cells, o.
oxalate
    plasma, o.

oxalemia
oxamniquine (Vansil)
oxamyristic acid
oxidized hemoglobin
oximeter
    ear o.
    finger o.
oximetry
oxonemia
oxophenarsine
oxygen (O2)
    -hemoglobin dissociation curve, o.
    saturation, o.
    transport, o.
oxygenated
    hemoglobin, o.
oxygenation
oxyhematin
oxyhematoporphyrin
oxyheme
oxyhemochromogen
oxyhemoglobin
oxyhemoglobinometer
oxyhemogram
oxyhemograph
oxyhyperglycemia
oxymyoglobin
oxyphenbutazone
oxyphilic erythroblasts
Oxytrak pulse oximeter
Oz
    allotypes, O.
    antigen, O.
    isotypic determinant, O.
ozone

Additional entries

P

P blood group
P24
   antibody, P.
   antigen, P.
   antigen capture assay, P.
PABA (p-aminobenzoic acid)
pachyemia
packed
   cell volume, p. (PCV)
   field, p.
   marrow, p.
   red cells, p. (PRC)
PaCO2 (partial pressure of carbon dioxide in arterial blood)
PAF (platelet-activating factor)
   -acether, P.
Pageblot system
Paget's disease
pagophagia
PAIDS (pediatric AIDS)
painful bruising syndrome
pale thrombus
palindrome
palindromic
pallid
pallor
p-aminobenzoic acid (PABA)
PAN (polyarteritis nodosa)
panagglutinable
panagglutination
panagglutinin
Panax ginseng
pancreas
pancreatic oncofetal antigen (POA)
pancreatitis
pancytopenia
Pander's islands
panhematopenia
panhematopoietic
panhemocytophthis
Panheprin
panimmunity
panleukopenia virus
panlymphopenia
Panton-Valentine leukocidin
Panwarfin
pan-cultured
PAP (peroxidase-antiperoxidase)
   immunoperoxidase, P.
papain
paperadioimmunosorbent test (PRIST)
papilledema
papillomavirus
Papovaviridae
papovavirus
pappataci fever virus
Pappenheimer bodies
papular
papule
papulomacular
para-aminosalicylic acid
paracoccidioidomycosis
Paragon immunofixation electrophoresis
parahemophilia
parahormone
parainfluenza
   antibody test, p.
   virus, p.
parallel
   plate dialyzer, p.
   track, p.
paramacular
paramomycin
paramyxovirus
Parana virus
paraneoplastic leukemoid reaction
parapertussis
paraphernalia
paraphilia
paraphiliac
parapneumonia
parapoxvirus
paraproctitis
paraprotein
   spike, p.
paraproteinemia

pararectal
parasexuality
parasitemia
parasite
parasitic
   thrombus, p.
parasitologic
parathyroid
parathyroidectomy
paratope
paratyphoid
   agglutination, p.
   fever, p.
   immunization, p.
paravaccinia
paravirus
parenteral
parietal thrombus
Parodi-Irgens sarcoma virus
parotitis
parovirus
paroxysm
paroxysmal
   cold hemoglobinuria, p. (PCH)
   nocturnal hemoglobinuria, p. (PNH)
parrot virus
partial
   antigen, p.
   exchange transfusion, p.
   thromboblastin time, p. (PTT)
partner
   notification, p.
Parvoviridae
parvovirus
PAS (peripheral access system OR periodic acid-Schiff)
   orange G, P.
   port, P.
   reagent, P.
   stain, P.
Paschen bodies
PASG (pneumatic anti-shock garment)
passenger leukocytes
passive
   agglutination, p.
   cutaneous anaphylaxis, p. (PCA)

passive *(continued)*
   hemagglutination, p.
   immunity, p.
   immunotherapy, p.
Passovoy factor
Pasteur
   effect, P.
   theory, P.
Pasteurella
pasteurellosis
pasteurization
   theory, p.
pasteurized Factor VIII concentrate
pathergy
pathoclisis
pathogen
pathogenesis
pathogenicity
pathognomonic
pathologic leukocytosis
pathway
pauciarticular
Paul-Bunnell test
Paul-Bunnell-Davidsohn test
pavementing
PBI (protein-bound iodine)
PBLs (peripheral blood lymphocytes)
PBMC (peripheral blood mononuclear cells)
PBV (predicted blood volume)
PCA (passive cutaneous anaphylaxis)
PCA-1 antigen
P. carinii (Pneumocystis carinii)
PC-55
PCH (paroxysmal cold hemoglobinuria)
PCNA (proliferating cell nuclear antigen)
pCO2 (carbon dioxide pressure)
PCP (Pneumocystis carinii pneumonia)
PCR (polymerase chain reaction)
PCT (prothrombin consumption time)
PCV (packed cell volume)
PDGF (platelet-derived growth factor)
peak
   -and-trough levels, p.
   blood flow, p.
pediatric AIDS (PAIDS)

Pedvax HIB
pefloxacin
PEG (polyethylene glycol)
    IL-2, P. (polyethylene glycolated IL-2)
pegademase bovine
Pel-Ebstein fever
pelgeroid
Pelger-Huet
    anomaly, P.
    cells, P.
pemphigoid
pemphigus
    vulgaris, p.
PEN (pharmacy equivalent name)
penectomy
penicillin
    G, p.
penicillinase-producing Neisseria
    gonorrhoeae (PPNG)
penicilloic acid
penicilloylpolylysine
penile
    ring, p.
penis
penitis
pentagastrin
Pentam 300
pentamidine
    aerosolization, p.
    isethionate, p.
    spray, p.
pentosan polysulfate (PPS)
pentose phosphate
    pathway, p.
    shunt, p.
peptide
    hormone, p.
    synthetase, p.
    T, p.
peptidoglycan
peptone plasma
peptonemia
Peptostreptococcus
per anum
per os
per rectum

Percoll technique
percutaneous needle biopsy
perfluorochemical
perforin
perfused
perfusion
    pump, p.
perfusionist
perianal
    herpes, p.
pericyte
Peridex
perihepatitis
periodic acid-Schiff stain (PAS)
perioral cyanosis
peripheral
    access system, p. (PAS)
    blood, p.
    blood lymphocytes, p. (PBLs)
    blood mononuclear cells, p. (PBMC)
    circulation, p.
    cyanosis, p.
    nervous system, p. (PNS)
    smear, p.
periphery
peripolesis
periportal
perirectal
perithelial
    cell, p.
periwinkle plant
perleche
permeability
permeable
pernicious anemia
peroxidase
    -antiperoxidase, p. (PAP)
    hemolysis, p.
    reaction, p.
    -staining cytoplasmic granules, p.
Peroxyl
persistent generalized lymphadenopathy
    (PGL)
Pertscan 99m
pertussis
    immune globulin, p.

pertussis *(continued)*
   toxin, p.
   vaccine, p.
pessary cell
petechiae
petechial
Petri dish
Peyer's patches
PF4 (platelet factor 4)
PFGE (pulsed field gradient gel electrophoresis)
Pfieffer's
   disease, P.
   phenomenon, P.
Pfiffner and Myers' method
PFS (primary fibromyalgia syndrome)
PGL (persistent generalized lymphadenopathy)
pH (hydrogen ion concentration)
PHA (phytohemagglutinin antigen)
phage
   typing, p.
phagedenic
phagocytable
phagocyte
phagocytic
   activity, p.
   assay, p.
   cell, p.
   defenses, p.
   index, p.
   thrombus, p.
phagocytin
phagocytize
phagocytoblast
phagocytolysis
phagocytolytic
phagocytose
phagocytosis
phagocytotic
phagokaryosis
phagological
phagolysis
phagolysosome
phagolytic
phagosome

phagotype
phallectomy
phallic
phalliform
phallitis
phalloplasty
phallus
pharmacogenetic
pharmacokinetic
pharmacy equivalent name (PEN)
pharmokinetic
pharyngeal
   herpes, p.
   pouch syndrome, p.
pharyngoconjunctival fever virus
Phase I, II, III studies
phase-specific
phased array
phasein
phasin
phenethicillin potassium
phenolemia
phenotype
phenotypic
phenotyping
phenprocoumon
phenylbutazone
phenylhydrazine anemia
pheresis
Philadelphia chromosome
Philippine
   dengue, P.
   hemorrhagic fever, P.
phlebitis
PHK (platelet phosphohexokinase)
PHLA (postheparin lipolytic activity)
phlebitic
phlebitis
phleboclysis
phlebogram
phlebolith
phleborrhagia
phleborrhexis
phlebostasis
phlebostenosis
phlebothrombosis

phlebotome
phlebotomize
Phlebotomus
 argentipes, P.
 chinensis. P.
 papatasii. P.
 sergenti, P.
 verrucarum, P.
phlebotomus fever
phlebotomy
phlogocyte
phlogocytosis
phloxine-tartrazine stain
Phoma
phorbol ester
phosphatase
phosphate-buffered saline
phosphatemia
phosphatidylcholine
phosphatidylethanolamine
phosphatidylinositol-specific phospholipase C (PIPLC)
phospholipase
phospholipid
phospholipidemia
phosphomonoesterase
phosphonoformate
phosphonoformic acid
phosphoribosyl pyrophosphate
phosphorothioate analogue
phosphorylase
phosphorylate
phosphorylation
Phosphotope oral solution
phosphotransferase
photohemotachometer
photomethemoglobin
photophoresis
phthisis
phylloquinone
phylogenetic
physiologic
 anemia, p.
 hypogammaglobulinemia, p.
 leukocytosis, p.
 salt solution, p. (PSS)

phytoanaphylactogen
phytohemagglutinin antigen (PHA)
phytonadione
phytoprecipitin
phytosensitinogen
pica
Pichinde virus
picibanil (OK-432)
Pick's cells
pickwickian syndrome
picodnavirus
picogram
picornavirus
PID (plasma iron disappearance)
PIDT (plasma iron disappearance time)
piggybacking
pine cone extract
ping-ponging
pinocytosis
pion therapy
pionemia
PIPLC (phosphatidylinositol-specific
 phospholipase C)
pipobroman
piritrexim isoethionate
piroplasmosis
Piry virus
PIT (plasma iron turnover)
Pitkin menstruum
PITR (plasma iron turnover rate)
Pittsburgh pneumonia agent
pituitary basophilism
pityriasis
PKD (pyruvinate kinase deficiency)
PKV (killed poliomyelitis vaccine)
PLA I
 antigen, P.
placebo
 alum preparation, p.
 -controlled study, p.
 -effect, p.
placental
 blood flow, p.
 oxygenation, p.
 transfusion, p.
plague

plague *(continued)*
  serum, p.
  toxin, p.
  vaccine, p.
plakins
plaque
  -forming cell assay, p.
Plasbumin
plasma
  albumose p.
  antihemophilic human p.
  blood p.
  citrated p.
  expanded p.
  fresh frozen p.
  hyperimmune p.
  lymph p.
  muscle p.
  normal human p.
  oxalate p.
  peptone p.
  pooled p.
  salt p.
  true p.
plasma acid phosphatase
plasma activation
plasma alteration
plasma cell
  antigen, p.
  leukemia, p.
plasma clotting time
plasma dyscrasia
plasma exchange
plasma expander
plasma half-life
plasma hemoglobin
plasma iron
  clearance, p. (PIC)
  clearance half-time, p.
  disappearance, p. (PID)
  disappearance time, p. (PIDT)
  turnover, p. (PIT)
  turnover rate, p. (PITR)
plasma kallikrein
plasma membrane
plasma protein

plasma protein fraction
plasma recalcification
plasma renin activity
plasma skimming
plasma substitute
plasma-thrombin clot method
plasma thromboplastin (PT)
  antecedent, p. (PTA) — factor XI
  clearance, p. (PTC)
  component, p. (PTC) — factor XI
plasma transfusion
plasma triglyceride
plasma volume
  expander, p.
  extender, p.
plasmablast
plasmacrit
plasmacyte
plasmacytic
  leukemia, p.
  series, p.
plasmacytoid
  lymphocyte, p.
plasmacytoma
plasmacytosis
plasmagene
plasmal
plasmalogen
Plasmalyte
Plasmanate
plasmapheresis
Plasma-Plex
Plasmatein
plasmatherapy
plasmatic
plasmid
plasmin
  coagulation, p.
plasminogen
  activator, p.
plasmocyte
Plasmodium
  vivax, P.
plasmoma
plasmonucleic acid
plate

plate *(continued)*
   thrombosis, p.
   thrombus, p.
platelet
   -activating factor, p. (PAF)
   adhesiveness, p.
   agglutination, p.
   agglutinin, p.
   aggregation test, p.
   antigen, p.
   autoantibodies, p.
   clumping, p.
   clustering, p.
   count, p.
   defect, p.
   -derived growth factor, p. (PDGF)
   factor, p.
   fibrinogen, p.
   -free plasma, p.
   isoantibodies, p.
   membrane-bound IgG, p.
   nadir, p.
   peroxidase, p.
   phosphohexokinase, p. (PHK)
   -poor blood, p.
   -poor plasma, p.
   retention test, p.
   -rich blood, p.
   -rich plasma, p.
   survival test, p.
   suspension immunofluorescence test, p. (PSIFT)
   thrombosis, p.
   thrombus, p.
   transfusion, p.
plateletpheresis
plating
pleiotropic
   genes, p.
pleocytosis
pleokaryocyte
pleomorphic
pleomorphism
pleonectic
pleonexia
pleotropia

pleuropneumonia-like organisms (PPLO)
plotolysin
plototoxin
PLT (primed lymphocyte typing)
Plummer-Vinson syndrome
pluriresistant
plus-stranded RNA genome virus
PLV (live poliomyelitis vaccine)
PMB (polymorphonuclear basophil)
PME (polymorphonuclear eosinophil)
PML (progressive multifocal leukoencephalopathy)
PMN (polymorphonuclear neutrophil)
PMR (polymyalgia rheumatica)
pneumathemia
pneumatic anti-shock garment (PASG)
pneumobacillus
pneumococcal
   polysaccharide, p.
   vaccine, p.
pneumococcemia
pneumococci
pneumococcus (pneumococci)
pneumocystic
Pneumocystis carinii (P. carinii)
   carinii pneumonia, P. (PCP)
pneumocystis
   pneumonia, p.
   pneumonitis, p.
pneumocystosis
pneumoenteritis
pneumohemia
pneumolysin
pneumonemia
pneumonia
pneumonic
pneumonitis
Pneumopent
Pneumovax
   23. P.
pneumovirus
PNH (paroxysmal nocturnal hemoglobinuria)
   cell, P.
PNI (psychoneuroimmunology)
PNS (peripheral nervous system)

pO2 (oxygen partial pressure)
POA (pancreatic oncofetal antigen)
Pohl's test
poietin
poikiloblast
poikilocyte
poikilocythemia
poikilocytosis
poikilothrombocyte
poin
Poiseuille's
   law, P.
   space, P.
pokeroot
pokeweed mitogen (PWM)
pol gene
polar anemia
polio (poliomyelitis)
   vaccine hyperimmunization, p.
poliocidal
polioclastic
polioencephalitis
polioencephalomyelitis
polioencephalopathy
polioencephalotropic
polioencephlomeningomyelitis
poliomyelencephalopathy
poliomyeliticidal
poliomyelitis
   vaccine, p.
   virus, p.
poliomyelopathy
poliovirus
   muris, p.
pollen
   antigen, p.
pollenogenic
pollinosis
poly (polymorphonuclear leukocyte)
poly I:C (polyriboinosinic:polyribocytidylic)
polyacrylamide gel
polyagglutination
polyarteritis
   nodosa, p. (PAN)
polyarthritis

polyarticular
polychemotherapy
polychondritis
polychromasia
polychromatic
   erythroblast, p.
   erythrocyte, p.
polychromatophil
   cell, p.
polychromatophilia
polychromatophilic
   erythrocyte, p.
polychromatosis
polychromemia
polyclonal
   antibodies, p.
   hypergammaglobulinemia, p.
   hyperglobulinemia, p.
polycyte
polycythemia
   appropriate p.
   benign p.
   compensatory p.
   hypertonica, p.
   inappropriate p.
   myelopathic p.
   primary p.
   rubra, p.
   rubra vera, p.
   secondary p.
   splenomegalic p.
   spurious p.
   stress p.
   vera, p.
polydrug
   abuse, p.
   therapy, p.
polyemia
   polycythaemica, p.
polyendocrine autoimmune disease
polyethylene
   glycol, p.
   glycolated IL-2, p. (PEG IL-2)
polyhemia
polyimmunoglobulin
polyinfection

polylymphocytic
   leukemia, p.
polylysine
polymer
polymerase
   chain reaction, p. (PCR)
polymerid
polymerism
polymerization
polymicrobial
polymicrobic
polymorphism
polymorphocyte
polymorphonuclear
   basophil, p. (PMB)
   eosinophil, p. (PME)
   leukocyte, p.
   neutrophil, p. (PMN)
polymyalgia
   arteritica, p.
   rheumatica, p. (PMR)
polymyelencephalitis
polymyositis
polyneuritis
polyneuropathy
polynucleotide
   ligase, p.
   nucleotidyltransferase, p.
   phosphorylase, p.
polyomavirus
polypeptide
polypeptidemia
polypharmaceutic
polypharmacy
polyphyletic theory
polyploid
polyriboinosinic:polyribocytidylic (poly I:C)
polysaccharide
polysaccharose
polyserositis
polysubstance abuse
polyvalent
   allergy, p.
   serum, p.
   vaccine, p.

pompholyhemia
Pongola virus
pooled
   blood, p.
   plasma, p.
   serum, p.
pooling
popin
popper (amyl nitrite)
porphobilinogen
porphyria
   erythropoietica, p.
porphyrin
porphyrinemia
porphyrinogen
port
Port-A-Cath
portacaval shunt
portal
   circulation, p.
   hypertension, p.
portosystemic
postalbumin
posthemorrhagic anemia
postheparin lipolytic activity (PHLA)
postirradiation syndrome
postperfusion syndrome
postprandial blood sugar (PPBS)
postpump syndrome
posttransfusion
   AIDS, p.
   hepatitis, p.
   mononucleosis, p.
   syndrome, p.
postvaccinal
postvaccinial
postzone
potassemia
potassium
potentialization
potentiation
potentiator
Powassan virus
pox
poxvirus
PPBS (postprandial blood sugar)

PPD (purified protein derivative)
PPD-S (purified protein derivative-standard)
PPLO (pleuropneumonia-like organisms)
PPNG (penicillinase-producing Neisseria gonorrhoeae)
PPS (pentosan polysulfate)
Pr antigen
Prausnitz-Kustner
    antibodies, P.
    reaction, P.
PRC (packed red cells)
pre-B
    acute lymphocytic leukemia, p.
    cell, p.
Precef
precipitable
    antibody, p.
precipitate
precipitation
precipitin
    curve, p.
    reaction, p.
    ring, p.
precipitinogen
precipitinoid
precipitophore
precipitum
precursor
Pred-G-SOP
predicted blood volume (PBV)
predictive value
prednimustine
prednisolone
prednisone
preeclampsia
preeclamptic
    toxemia, p.
preelacin
pregnancy serum
pregnant mare's serum
prekallikrein
preleukemia
preleukemic
premonocyte
premunition

premunitive
premyeloblast
premyelocyte
Pre-Pen
pressure point
pre-T cell
    acute lymphocytic leukemia, p.
prezone
primaquine
    -sensitive anemia, p.
primary
    anemia, p.
    bubo, p.
    fibromyalgia syndrome, p. (PFS)
    immune response, p.
    immunodeficiency, p.
    splenic panhematopenia, p.
    thrombus, p.
primed lymphocyte typing (PLT)
primethamine
primitive
    erythroblasts, p.
    white cells, p.
prion
PRIST (paperadioimmunosorbent test)
private antigens
pro time (prothrombin time)
proaccelerin
proactivator
proagglutinoid
proantithrombin
probenecid
Probit analysis
procoagulant
procollagen
procollagenase
proconvertin (factor VII)
Procrit
proctalgia
proctitis
    obliterans, p.
proctocolitis
proctogenic
Procytox
prodromal
prodrome

production-defect anemia
proerythroblast
proerythrocyte
profibrinolysin
progenitor
progeny
prognostic marker
progranulocyte
progranulocytic
   leukemia, p.
progressive
   multifocal leukoencephalopathy, p.
     (PML)
   thrombus, p.
Project Inform
prokallikrein
prokaryote
Proleukin
proleukocyte
proliferating cell nuclear antigen (PCNA)
proline
prolonged
   bleeding time, p.
   coagulation time, p.
prolymphocyte
prolymphocytic
   leukemia, p.
PRO-MACE/MOPP
promegakaryocyte
promegaloblast
promiscuity
promiscuous
promonocyte
promyelocyte
promyelocytic leukemia
pronormoblast
properdin
propagated thrombus
propagating thrombosis
prophylactic
   serum, p.
prophylax
prophylaxed
prophylaxis
propiolactone
propionicacidemia

proplasmacyte
Proplex
propolis
Prosorba Column
prospective study
prostacyclin
prostaglandin
prostate-specific antigen (PSA)
prostitute
prostitution
protamine sulfate
protease
proteid
proteidic
proteidogenous
protein
   A column, p.
   -A-peroxidase conjugate im-
     munoperoxidase, p.
   -bound iodine, p. (PBI)
   C, p.
   -deficiency anemia, p.
   electrophoresis, p.
   -glutamine, p.
   kinase, p.
   kinase C, p.
   -losing enteropathy, p.
   quotient, p.
   S, p.
   spike, p.
   synthesis, p.
proteinaceous
proteinase
proteinemia
proteinuria
Protenate
proteoglycan
proteolysis
proteolytic
   enzyme, p.
Proteus
   mirabilis, P.
   vulgaris, P.
prothrombin (factor II)
   consumption time, p. (PCT)
   -converting principal, p.

prothrombin (factor II) *(continued)*
    time, p. (PT)
prothrombinase
prothrombinogen
prothrombinogenic
prothrombinokinase
prothrombinopenia
protide
protidemia
protocol
    019, p.
protoheme
protohemin
protoleukocyte
proton
protoporphyria
protoporphyrin
protoporphyrinogen oxidase
protozoa
protozoan
    enteritis, p.
protransglutamase
proviral
provirus
provocation typhoid
Prowazek's bodies
Prowazek-Greeff bodies
Prower factor
proxicromil
prozonal
prozone
Prussian blue reaction
PSA (prostate-specific antigen)
Pseudallescheria
    boydii, P.
pseudoagglutination
pseudoallele
pseudoallergic
    reaction, p.
pseudoallergy
pseudoanaphylaxis
pseudoanemia
pseudobacillus
pseudobacterium
pseudocowpox virus
pseudogene

pseudoglobulin
pseudohemagglutination
pseudohemophilia
pseudohemoptysis
pseudohermaphrodite
pseudohermaphroditism
pseudohypericin
pseudohyperkalemia
pseudohyphae
pseudohyponatremia
pseudoicterus
pseudoinfectious
    proctitis, p.
pseudojaundice
pseudo-Kaposi syndrome
pseudoleukemia
pseudoleukocythemia
pseudolymphoma
pseudomethemogloblin
pseudomonal
    toxin, p.
Pseudomonas
    aeruginosa, P.
    fluorescens, P.
    maltophilia, P.
    pickettii, P.
    stutzeri, P.
pseudomycelia
pseudoreaction
pseudoremission
PSIFT (platelet suspension immunofluorescence test)
psittacosis
psoralen
psoriasis
psoriatic
    arthritis, p.
PSS (physiological salt solution)
psychological sex
psychoneuroimmunology (PNI)
Psychotonin M
PT (plasma thromboplastin OR prothrombin time)
PTA (plasma thromboplastin antecedent—factor XI)

PTC (plasma thromboplastin clearance or
 component)
ptomainemia
PTT (partial thromboplastin time)
P24
   antibody, P.
   antigen, P.
   antigen capture assay, P.
public antigen
PUF (pure ultrafiltration)
Pullularia
pulsed field gradient gel electrophoresis
 (PFGE)
pump-oxygenator
pure
   leukocytosis, p.
   red cell agenesis, p.
   red cell anemia, p.
   red cell aplasia, p.
   ultrafiltration, p. (PUF)
purified protein derivative (PPD)
   -standard, p. (PPD-S)
purine nucleoside phosphorylase
purinemia
puromycin
purpura
   fulminans, p.
purpuric
Purtillo lymphoproliferative syndrome
pus cell
pustulosis
   vacciniformis acuta, p.
   varioliformis acuta, p.
PWA (person with AIDS)
PWARC (person with ARC)
PWM (pokeweed mitogen)

pycnemia
pyemia
pyknemia
pyknocyte
pyknocytosis
pyknotic
   bodies, p.
pyoderma
   gangrenosum, p.
pyogenic
   arthritis, p.
pyosapremia
pyosepticemia
pyostomatitis
pyotoxinemia
pyrantel pamoate
pyrazinamide
pyrenemia
pyretherapy
pyretic therapy
pyretotherapy
pyridoxilated stroma-free hemoglobin
pyridoxine
   -responsive anemia, p.
pyrimethamine-sulfadoxine
pyrimidine
pyrogen
pyroglobulin
pyroglobulinemia
pyrophosphate
Pyrost
pyruvate kinase
   deficiency, p. (PKD)
pyruvemia
pyruvic acid

Additional entries

Q fever
QA antigen
Q-banding (quinacrine banding)
QT6 cell line
qualitative clot retraction
quanti-Pirquet
   reaction, q.
   test, q.
quantitation
quantitative
Quaranfil virus
quarantine
   period, q.
quarantined
quaternary
Quell
quellung reaction

quenching
   fluorescent q.
quercetin
   -3-rutinoside, q.
Queyrat's erythroplasia
Quick's test
quiescent
quinacrine
   banding, q. Q-banding)
   hydrochloride, q.
Quinamm
quinine
Quinton-Mahurkar dual-lumen catheter
Quin-2
quotidian fever
quotient

Additional entries

R

RA (rheumatoid arthritis)
    cell, R.
    latex fixation test, R.
    scan uptake, R.
rabbit
    -antidog thymus serum, r. (RADTS)
    -antimouse thymocyte, r. (RAMT)
    -antirat lymphocyte serum, r. (RARLS)
    fibroma virus, r.
    myxoma virus, r.
    papilloma virus, r.
rabid
rabies
    immune globulin, r.
    vaccine, r.
    virus, r.
rabiform
Rachromate-51
Racobalamin
rad (radiation-absorbed dose)
radial immunodiffusion (RID)
    assay, r. (RIDA)
radian
radiation
    absorbed dose, r. (rad)
    leukemia virus, r. (RadLV)
    syndrome, r.
    therapy, r.
radioactive
    colloidal gold, r.
    gold, r.
    iodinated human serum albumin, r. (RIHSA)
    iodinated serum albumin, r. (RISA)
    iodine, r. (RAI)
    iodine uptake, r. (RAIU)
    label, r.
    tracer, r.
    uptake, r. (RAU)
radioallergosorbent
    test, r. (RAST)
radiocarcinogenesis
radiocobalt-labeled vitamin B-12
radiodilution
radioenzyme
radioenzymatic
    assay, r. (REA)
radiogold
radioimmune
    precipitation, r.
radioimmunity
radioimmunoassay (RIA)
radioimmunodetection (RAID)
radioimmunodiffusion
radioimmunoelectrophoresis
radioimmunoprecipitation (RIP)
    assay, R. (RIPA)
radioimmunosorbent
    test, R. (RIST)
radioiodine (I131)
radioiron
radioisotope
radioisotopic
radiolabeled
    probe, r.
radioligand
    assay, r.
radiomutation
radion
radionuclide
radiopharmaceutical
radiopharmacy
radiophosphorus
radiopotassium
radiopotentiation
radiopraxis
radioprotective
radioreceptor
    assay, r. (RRA)
radioresistant
radiosensitive
radiotherapy
radiotoxemia
radium
RadLV (radiation leukemia virus)

RADTS (rabbit-antidog thymus serum)
ragocyte
    cell, r.
ragweed allergen
RAI (radioactive iodine)
    scan, R.
    scan uptake, R.
RAID (radioimmunodetection)
RAIU (radioactive iodine uptake)
Rai's stage
Raji cell assay
Ramon flocculation
RAMT (rabbit-antimouse thymocyte)
random
    blood sugar, r.
    controlled trial, r.
    platelets, r.
randomization
randomize
rapid plasma reagin (RPR)
RARLS (rabbit-antirat lymphocyte serum)
Rasheed sarcoma virus
RAST (radioallergosorbent test)
    inhibition assay, R.
Rastafarian cult
rat
    thymus antiserum, r.
    virus, r.
RAU (radioactive uptake)
Rauscher
    leukemia, R.
    leukemia virus, R,
RAV (Rous-associated virus)
Raynaud's
    phenomenon, R.
    sign, R.
RBC (red blood cell OR red blood count)
RBC/hpf (red blood cells per high-power field)
RBCIT (red blood cell iron turnover)
RBCM (red blood cell mass)
RCC (red cell count)
rCD4-IgG
RCF (red cell folate)
RCIA (red cell immune adherence)
RCM (red cell mass)
RCV (red cell volume)
RDDP (RNA-dependent DNA polymerase)
RDE (receptor-destroying enzyme)
RDRV (Rhesus diploid cell strain rabies vaccine)
RDW (red cell diameter width)
REA (radioenzymatic assay)
reactive
    arthritis, r.
    hyperemia blood flow, r. (RHBF)
reactivity
reagent
reagin
reaginic antibody
Rebuck's skin window technique
recalcification time
recall antigen
recent thrombus
receptor
    destroying enzyme, r.- (RDE)
recessive
    gene, r.
    trait, r.
recipient
reciprocal gene
reciprocation
recognin
recombinant
    alpha interferon, r.
    DNA, r.
    human beta interferon, r.
    human erythropoietin, r. (rHuEPO)
    human granulocyte colony stimulating factor, r. (rGM-CSF)
    immunoblot assay, r.
    murine granulocyte-macrophage colony-stimulating factor, r. (rmGM-CSF)
    soluble CD4, r. (T4)
    tissue plasminogen activator, r. (rt-PA)
    vector, r.
recombination
recombinational germline theory
Recombivax

recreational
  drug, r.
  sex, r.
recrement
recrementitious
recruitment factor
rectal
  fisting, r.
  gonorrhea, r.
  intercourse, r.
  penetration, r.
  sex, r.
  trauma, r.
rectitis
rectocolitis
rectum
red blood cell (RBC)
  iron turnover, r. (RBCIT)
  mass, r. (RBCM)
  survival, r.
red blood cells per high-power field (RBC/hpf)
red blood count (RBC)
red cell
  aplasia, r.
  casts, r.
  coating, r.
  count, r. (RCC)
  diameter width, r. (RCDW)
  folate, r. (RCF)
  fragility, r.
  ghost, r.
  immune adherence, r. (RCIA)
  indices, r.
  mass, r. (RCM)
  morphology, r.
  sizing, r.
  volume, r. (RCV)
red marrow
red thrombus
red venous blood
Redisol
reduced hemoglobin
reducing agent
reductase
redwater disease

Redy 2000 hemodialysis system
Reed cell
Reed-Sternberg giant cell
reference strain
refractory sideroblastic anemia
regenerative shift
regional lymph nodes
regulator gene
Reider
  cell leukemia, R.
  lymphocyte, R.
Reilly bodies
reinoculation
Reiter
  protein complement-fixation, R. (RCPF)
  protein complement-fixation test, R. (RPCFT)
  syndrome, R.
  treponemes, R.
Reitman-Frankel test
relative
  leukocytosis, r.
  polycythemia, r.
releasing factor
Relia-Vac
remission
Rendu-Osler-Weber disease
renin substrate
reovirus
repeated DNA sequences
replacement transfusion
replicate
replication
replicative vaccine
replicon
repressed gene
repressor
  gene, r.
reptilase
  time, r.
RES (reticuloendothelial system)
reservoir of virus
resistance
  -inducing factor, r.
  transfer factor, r. (RTF)

resistant
   strain, r.
resorbed
resorption
Respigard II nebulizer
respiratory
   acidosis, r.
   syncytial, r. (RS)
   syncytial virus, r. (RSV)
resting
   hase, r.
   potential, r.
   T-cells, r.
restitope
restriction fragment length polymorphism (RFLP)
retic (reticulocyte)
   count, r. (reticulocyte count)
reticular cells
reticulin staining
reticulocyte
   count, r.
   production index, r. (RPI)
reticulocytogenic
reticulocytopenia
reticulocytosis
reticuloendothelial
   blockade, r.
   cell leukemia, r.
   system, r. (RES)
reticuloendothelioma
reticuloendotheliosis
reticulohistiocytary
reticulohistiocytoma
reticulohistiocytosis
reticuloid
reticuloma
reticulopenia
reticulosarcoma
Reticulose
reticulosis
reticulum cell
   sarcoma, r.
retinal ischemia
Retrogen
retrospective study

Retrovir
retroviral
retrovirology
retrovirus
   replication, r.
rev (regulator of expression of virion proteins)
reverse
   genetics, r.
   passive Arthus reaction, r.
   transcriptase, r.
   transcriptase inhibitors, r.
Reye's syndrome
RF (rheumatoid factor)
R-51211
RFLA (rheumatoid factor-like activity)
RFLP (restriction fragment length polymorphism)
RG 12915
rGM-CSF (recombinant human granulocyte colony stimulating factor)
rgpl 60
Rh (Rhesus)
   agglutinin, R.
   antibody, R.
   antigen, R.
   antiserum, R.
   blood group, R.
   factor, R.
   genes, R.
   immune globulin, R.
   immunization, R.
   incompatibility, R.
   isoantigen, R.
   isoimmunization, R.
Rh-negative
Rh-null syndrome
Rh-positive
rhabdocyte
rhabdoid
rhabdovirus
Rhadotorula
rhagiocrine cell
RHBF (reactive hyperemia blood flow)
Rheinberg microscope
rheology

rhestocythemia
Rhesus (Rh)
    diploid cell strain rabies vaccine, R. (RDRV)
    factor, R.
    macaque, R
    rotavirus vaccine, R. (RRV)
rheumatic factor
rheumatoid
    arthritis, r. (RA)
    factor, r. (RF)
    factor-like activity, r. (RFLA)
rheumatologic
Rheumatrex
rhinoviral
rhinovirus
Rho(D) immune globulin
rhodamine isothiocyanate
RhoGAM immune globulin
rhopheocytosis
rHuEPO (recombinant human erythropoietin)
RIA (radioimmunoassay)
RIBA-HIV
ribavirin
Ribbert's thrombosis
riboflavin
ribonuclear protein (RNP)
ribonuclease (RNAse)
ribonucleic acid (RNA)
ribonucleoprotein
ribose
ribosome
ribozymes
Richettsia agglutination
Richter syndrome
ricin
rickets
rickettsemia
RID (radial immunodiffusion)
RIDA (radial immunodiffusion assay)
Ridaura
Rieder cell
    leukemia, R.
Rieder's lymphocyte
Rifabutin

rifabutine
rifampicin
rifampin
rifamycin
Rift Valley fever virus
right shift
RIHSA (radioactive iodinated human serum albumin)
rimantadine
rimming
Rindfleisch's cells
ringed sideroblasts
Ringer's lactate
RIP (radioimmunoprecipitation)
RIPA (radioimmunoprecipitation assay)
RISA (radioactive iodinated serum albumin)
risk
    behavior, r.
    factor, r.
risky sex
RIST (radioimmunosorbent test)
ristocetin cofactor test
RIT 4237
ritodrine
R-loop
rmGM-CSF (recombinant murine granulocyte-macrophage colony-stimulating factor)
RNA (ribonucleic acid)
    nucleotidyltransferase, R.
    polymerase, R.
    retrovirus, R.
    splicing, R.
    virus, R.
RNA-dependent DNA polymerase (RDDP)
RNA-directed DNA polymerase
RNA-directed RNA polymerase
RNAse (ribonuclease)
RNP (ribonuclear protein or ribonucleoprotein)
rocket immunoelectrophoresis
Rofcron A
Rollet's stroma
roll-tube culture

Romer's test
Rose-Waaler test
rosea-like
Rosenthal syndrome
rosette
    cell, r.
Rosewater's syndrome
Ross' bodies
rotavirus
Rotazyme
Roth's spots
Rotor's syndrome
Ro24-2027
Rouget cells
rouleau (pl. rouleaux)
    formation, r.
rouleaux (pl. of rouleau)
round cell
Rourke-Ernstein sedimentation rate
Rous
    -associated virus, R. (RAV)
    sarcoma virus, R. (RSV)
    test, R.
rovamycin
Rowasa enema
Roxanol CII
Roxanol Rescudose
Royal Free disease
RPCF (Reiter protein complement-fixation)
RPCFT (Reiter protein complement-fixation test)
RPI (reticulocyte production index)
RPR (rapid plasma reagin)
RRA (radioreceptor assay)
RRV (rhesus rotavirus vaccine)
RS (respiratory syncytial)
    virus, R.
RS-47
R64,633
rsT4
RSV (respiratory syncytial virus OR Rous sarcoma virus)
RTF (resistance transfer factor)
rt-PA (recombinant tissue plasminogen activator)
rubber (condom)
    dam, r.
rubella
    arthritis, r.
    titer, r.
    virus vaccine, r.
rubeola
Rubex
rubivirus
Rubner's test
Rubramin PC
Rubratope
rubriblast
rubricyte
Rumpel-Leede test
Runeberg's anemia
runting syndrome
Russell bodies
Russian spring-summer encephalitis virus
Rye classification

Additional entries

S

Sabin vaccine
Sabin-Feldman dye test
Sabouraud plate
Saccharomyces
SACE (serum angiotensin-converting enzyme)
SAE (sea algae extract)
safe sex
Sahli's method
SAIDS (simian AIDS)
saline
    agglutination, s.
    agglutinin, s.
    antibodies, s.
Salisbury common cold virus
saliva
    blot test, s.
    screening, s.
    spot test, s.
salivary
    -based assay, s.
    corpuscles, s.
    gland virus, s.
    virus, s.
salivation
salivatory
Salk vaccine
Salmonella
    choleraesuis, S.
    enteritidis, S.
Salmonella-Shigella agar
salmonella agglutinins
salmonella proctitis
salmonella serogroup D
salmonellal
salmonellosis
salt
    agglutination, s.
    plasma, s.
salted out
salvarsanized serum
Salzman test
San Joaquin valley fever

sandfly fever
Sandhoff's disease
Sandimmune
Sandostatin
sandwich technique
sanguicolous
sanguifacient
sanguiferous
sanguification
sanguimotor
sanguine
sanguineous
sanguinolent
sanguinopoietic
sanguinopurulent
sanguinoserous
sanguirenal
sanguis
sanguivorous
Santyl
SaO2 (arterial oxygen saturation)
saphhism
sarcoid
    arthritis, s.
sarcoidosis
sarcoma
sarcomagenic
sarcomatosis
sarcomatous
satellite
    lesion, s.
    virus, s.
satyriasis
satyromania
saxitoxin
SB (secondary B-cell)
SC (secretory component OR serum chemistry)
scalded skin syndrome
scanography
scarification
SCAT (sheep cell agglutination test)
scatemia

scavenger cell
SCG (serum chemistry graph)
SCH 39304
SCH 42427
Schaedler blood agar
Schalfijew's test
Schick test
Schiff test
Schilling
    blood count, S.
    classification, S.
    leukemia, S.
    test, S.
    -type monocytic leukemia, S.
schistocyte
schistocytosis
Schistosoma
schistosomiasis
schizocyte
schizont
Schlesinger's solution
Schonlein's disease
Schuffner's
    dots, S.
    stippling, S.
Schultz reaction
Schultz-Dale reaction
Schultze's granule masses
Schumm's test
Schwachman's syndrome
Schwachman-Diamond syndrome
Schwartzman's reaction
SCID (severe combined immunodeficiency)
scintigraphy
scintiphotography
scintiscan
Sclavo's serum
scleredema
sclerocythemia syndrome
sclerosant
sclerosis
sclerotherapy
sclerotic
scorbutic anemia
scorotemia

scrapie amyloid precursor protein
scratch test
Scribner shunt
SD (serologically defined OR streptodornase)
    antigen, S.
SDC-28
SDZ MSL-109
sea
    algae extract, s. (SAE)
    scurvy, s.
sea-blue histiocyte
secondary
    anemia, s.
    polycythemia, s.
    sex characteristics, s.
second-set
    phenomenon, s.
    rejection, s.
secretagogue
secreted immunoglobulin
secretor
secretory
    component, s. (SC)
    compound, s.
    IgA, s.
    immunoglobulin A, s.
    piece, s.
sed rate (sedimentation rate)
sedimentation
    coefficient, s.
    equilibrium, s.
    rate, s.
    time, s.
sedimentator
segmented
    cell, s.
    neutrophil, s.
segmenter
segs (segmented neutrophils)
Seidelin bodies
Selectomycin
Selenite F broth
selenoid cells
self
    -antigen, s.

self *(continued)*
   -fusion reaction, s.
   -infection, s.
   tolerance, s.
Seller's stain
semelincident
semen
seminal fluid
semipermeable
Semliki Forest virus
Semple vaccine
Semunya virus
semustine
Sendai virus
Sendoxan
Senear-Usher syndrome
sensitinogen
sensitivity
sensitization
sensitized
   cell, s.
   vaccine, s.
sensitizer
sensitizing
   antibodies, a.
sepiapterin reductase
septic
   anemia, s.
   arthritis, s.
   fever, s.
   shock, s.
septicemia
septicopyemia
Septra
Sequamycin
Sequence Multiple Analyzer (SMA)
sequential determinant
sequestered antigen
sequestration
sera (pl. of serum)
seralbumin
serial thrombin time (STT)
series
   aliphatic s.
   basophilic s.
   eosinophilic s.

series *(continued)*
   erythrocytic s.
   fatty s.
   granulocytic s.
   Hofmeister s.
   homologous s.
   leukocytic s.
   lymphocytic s.
   lyotropic s.
   monocytic s.
   myelocytic s.
   myeloid s.
   neutrophilic s.
   plasmacytic s.
   thrombocytic s.
serine proteinase
seroconversion
seroconvert
seroculture
serodefined
   antigen, s.
serodiagnosis
serofast
seroflocculation
seroglobulin
serogroup
seroimmunity
serolipase
serologic
   marker, s.
   test, s.
serological
   titer, s.
serologically defined (SD)
   antigen, s.
serology
   screen, s.
   test, s.
serolysin
seronegative
seronegativity
seropositive
seropositivity
seroprevalence
seroprevention
seroprognosis

seroprophylaxis
seroreaction
seroreactive
serorelapse
seroresistance
seroresistant
seroreversal
serorevertor
serosanguineous
serositis
serosurvey
serotherapy
serotonin
serotoxin
serotype
serous
serovaccination
serovar
serozyme
serpin
Serratia
   liquefaciens, S.
   marcescans, S.
   proteamaculans, S.
serum (pl. sera)
   active s.
   anallergenic s.
   anticholera s.
   anticomplementary s.
   anticrotalus s.
   antidiphtheritic s.
   antihepatic s.
   antilymphocyte s. (ALS)
   antimeningococcal s.
   antipertussis s.
   antiplague s.
   antiplatelet s.
   antipneumococcal s.
   antirabies s.
   antireticular cytotoxic s. (ACS)
   antiscarlatinal s.
   antistaphylococcal s.
   antistreptococcal s.
   antitetanic s. (ATS)
   antithymocyte s.
   antitoxic s.

serum *(continued)*
   antityphoid s.
   antivenomous s.
   bacteriolytic s.
   blood s.
   blood grouping s.
   convalescent s.
   cytotrophic s.
   despeciated s.
   endotheliolytic s.
   foreign s.
   heterologous s.
   homologous s.
   hyperimmune s.
   immune s.
   inactivated s.
   leukocytolytic s.
   Loffler's s.
   lymphatolytic s.
   monovalent s.
   motile s.
   nephrotoxic s.
   normal s.
   plague s.
   polyvalent s.
   pooled s.
   pregnancy s.
   pregnant mare's s.
   prophylactic s.
   salvarsanized s.
   Sclavo's s.
   specific s.
   streptococcus s.
   thyrotoxic s.
serum angiotensin-converting enzyme (SACE)
serum chemistry (SC)
   graph, s. (SCG)
   panel, s.
serum creatinine
serum electrolytes
serum-fast
serum ferritin
serum folate
   binder, s.
serum globulin

serum glutamate pyruvate transaminase (SGPT)
serum glutamic-oxaloacetic transaminase (SGOT)
serum hepatitis (SH)
    antigen, s.
serum iron
serum level
serum lytes
serum p24 antigen concentration
serum precipitable iodine
serum protein
    -bound iodine, s. (SPBI)
    electrophoresis, s. (SPEP)
serum prothrombin
    time, s.
    conversion accelerator, s. (SPCA)
serum rash
serum shock
serum sickness
serum thrombotic accelerator
serum urea nitrogen (SUN)
serum uric acid (SUA)
serumal
servomechanism
severe combined immunodeficiency (SCID)
sex
    assignment, s.
    change, s.
    chromatin, s.
    -conditioned, s.
    -conditioned gene, s.
    determination, s.
    differentiation, s.
    -influenced gene, s.
    -limited, s.
    -limited gene, s.
    limited protein, s.- (SLP)
    -linked, s.
    -linked agammaglobulinemia, s.
    -linked gene, s.
    orientation, s.
    perversion, s.
    reassignment, s.
    reversal, s.

sex *(continued)*
    -reversal gene, s.
    -reversal procedure, s.
sexual
    contact, s.
    deviant, s.
    deviation, s.
    dysfunction, s.
    exposure, s.
    identity, s.
    intercourse, s.
    orientation, s.
    partner, s.
    reassignment, s.
    sadism, s.
sexuality
sexually-transmitted disease (STD)
Sezary
    cell, S.
    syndrome, S.
SFHb (stroma-free hemoglobin)
7S gamma autoantibody
SGOT (serum glutamic-oxaloacetic transaminase)
SGPT (serum glutamate pyruvate transaminase)
SH (serum hepatitis)
    antigen, S.
shadow cell
Shaffer-Hartmann method
shake culture
shared needle
shedding
sheep
    cell agglutination test, s. (SCAT)
    erythrocytes, s.
    red blood cell, s. (SRBC)
sheet sign
shift
    to the left, s.
    to the right, s.
Shiga toxin
Shigella
    flexneri, s.
    sonnei, s.
shigella dysentery

shigellosis
shiitake
  extract, s.
  mushrooms, s.
Shine-Dalgarno sequence
shingles
shock
  antigen, s.
  blocks, s.
  syndrome, s.
shocky
Shohl's solution
shoot up
shooting gallery
short increment sensitivity index (SISI)
shortened
  bleeding time, s.
  coagulation time, s.
shotty nodes
shunt
  cyanosis, s.
shunting
SI (stimulation index)
Sia test
sialidase
sialophorin
sicca syndrome
sickle cell
  anemia, s.
  crisis, s.
  dactylitis, s.
  disease, s.
  -persistent fetal hemoglobin syn-
    drome, s.
  thalassemia, s.
  trait, s.
Sickledex reagent
sicklemia
sickling
side chain
  theory, s.
sideroachrestic anemia
sideroblast
sideroblastic
  anemia, s.
siderocyte

siderogenous
sideropenia
sideropenic
  anemia, s.
siderophage
siderophil
siderophilin
siderophilous
siderophore
siderosis
siderotic
  nodule, s.
siderous
SIg (cell-surface immunoglobulin)
Siga toxin
sigmavirus
signal sequence
silent gene
silicontungstate
Simbu virus
simian
  AIDS, s. (SAIDS)
  immunodeficiency virus, s. (SIV)
  sarcoma virus, s. (SSV)
  T-cell leukemia virus, s. (STLV)
  -type D retrovirus, s.
  virus, s. (SV)
Simon's septic factor
Simonsen phenomenon
Simplastin
simple achlorhydric anemia
simvastatin
Sindbis virus
single
  -agent chemotherapy, s.
  blind, s.
  -unit transfusion, s.
sinusoidal endothelial cell
Sips
  distribution, S.
  plot, S.
SIRS (soluble immune response suppressor)
SISI (short increment sensitivity index)
sissorexia
SIV (simian immunodeficiency virus)

sixth disease
Sjogren syndrome
SK (streptokinase)
    770 virus, S.
SK 38-39 (HIV-1 specific primer pair)
skeocytosis
skeptophylaxis
skin
    -fixed antibody, s.
    reactive factor, s.
    sensitizing antibodies, s.
    -specific histocompatibility antigen, s.
    test, s.
skinny needle
SKSD (streptokinase-streptodornase)
SL (streptolysin)
SLA (slide latex agglutination)
slaty anemia
SLE (systemic lupus erythematosus)
slim disease
slot blot technique
slow
    hemoglobin, s.
    reacting substance of anaphylaxis, s. (SRS-A)
    virus infection, s.
SLP (sex-limited protein)
sludged blood
sludging of blood
Sm (Smith) antigen
SMA (Sequence Multiple Analyzer)
    12 profile, S.
    12/60 profile, S.
    6/60 profile, S.
SMAC-23 series
SMAF (specific macrophage-arming factor)
smallpox
    vaccine, s.
Smith antigen
smoldering leukemia
smooth-rough variation
smudge cells
SMX/TMP (sulfamethoxazole/trimethoprim)
snapback DNA

snort (inhale drugs nasally)
Sn-proto porphyrin
social sex
sodium pertechnate Tc 99m
sodomist
sodomize
sodomy
soft sore
Solcotrans drainage/reinfusion system
solid-phase
    immunoabsorbent assay, s. (SPIA)
    immunoassay, s. (SPIA)
soluble
    CD4, s.
    immune response suppressor, s. (SIRS)
solvent-detergent method
Somacin formula
somatic
    agglutinin, s.
    antigen, s.
    mutation, s.
    O antigen, s.
somatomedin
somatostatin
somatotropic
somatotropin
Somogyi
    method, S.
    phenomenon, S.
    unit, S.
sorbic acid
sorter
Southern
    blot test, S.
    blotting, S.
spacer gel
Spanish fly
SPBI (serum protein-bound iodine)
SPCA (serum prothrombin conversion accelerator)
species
    immunity, s.
    specificity, s.
species-specific
    antigen, s.

species-specific *(continued)*
    immunity, s.
specific
    coagulation factor deficiency, s.
    immunity, s.
    macrophage arming factor, s. (SMAF)
    pathogen-free, s. (SPF)
    serum, s.
    suppressor cells, s.
specificity
specificness
spectinomycin
spectrin
spectrofluorometer
spectrofluorometry
spectrometer
spectrometry
spectrophotometer
spectrophotometry
spectroscope
spectroscopy
spectrotype
Spengler's fragment
SPEP (serum protein electrophoresis)
sperm
spermicidal
spermicide
spermine
    phosphate, s.
SPF (specific pathogen-free)
spherical
spherocyte
spherocytic
    serum, s.
spherocytosis
spheroplast
spherulin
sphingoglycolipid
sphingolipid
sphingolipidosis
sphingomyelinase
sphingophospholipid
SPIA (solid-phase immunoabsorbent assay or solid-phase immunoassay)
spiculated cells
spiculed RBC
spider
    angioma, s.
    telangiectasia, s.
    -web clot, s.
spinal fluid
    leukocyte counts.
    tap, s.
spindle cell
spindling
Spiractone
spiramycin
spiritual therapy
spirochetemia
spirochetes
spirochetosis
spirogermanium hydrochloride
spiromustine
spironolactone
spiroplatin
Spiro-32
splanchnic blood
spleen
splenectomize
splenectomy
splenemia
splenic anemia of infants
splenicterus
splenocaval shunt
splenocyte
splenohepatomegaly
splenomedullary leukemia
splenomegalic polycythemia
splenomegaly
splenomyelogenous leukemia
splenorenal shunt
splenorrhagia
split tolerance
split-virus vaccine
Spondweni virus
Spondylocladium
spontaneous agglutination
Sporothrix
    schenckii, S.
sporotrichosis
spreading factor
sprue

spruelike syndrome
spur cell
    anemia, s.
spurious polycythemia
SR (stimulation ratio)
SRBC (sheep red blood cell)
SRS-A (slow-reacting substance of anaphylaxis)
SS-A antigen
SS-B antigen
SSV (simian sarcoma virus)
stab (stabnuclear neutrophil)
    cell, s.
stable factor
stabnuclear neutrophil
staff
    cell, s.
    test, s.
staging of disease
stainable iron
Stammer's method
stanozolol
staph (staphylococcus)
    infection, s.
staphylocoagulase
staphylococcal
    protein A, s.
    protein A binding assay, s.
    toxin, s.
staphylococcemia
staphylococcic
staphylococcin
staphylococcosis
Staphylococcus
    aureus, S.
    epidermidis, S
    pyogenes, S.
    simulans, S.
staphylococcus clumping test
staphylohemia
staphylokinase
staphylolysin
Starling's hypothesis
starry-sky pattern
stave cells
STD (sexually-transmitted disease)

stem cell
    assay, s.
    leukemia, s.
    lymphoma, s.
    marrow, s.
Stemphyllium
sternal marrow aspiration
Sternberg's giant cells
Sternberg-Reed cells
Sterneedle test
steroid
    binding betaglobulin, s.
    dependence, s.
    -dependent, s.
steroidogenesis
Stevens-Johnson syndrome
Stewart-Treves syndrome
Still's disease
stimulation
    index, s. (SI)
    ratio, s. (SR)
stimulin
stimulon
stipple cell
stippling
St. John's wort
St. Louis encephalitis virus
STLV (simian T-cell leukemia virus)
stock culture
stomatitides (pl. of stomatitis)
stomatitis (pl. stomatitides)
stomatocace
stomatocyte
stomatocytosis
stomatoglossitis
stool
    culture, s.
    for O&P, s. (ova and parasites)
storage
    iron, s.
    pool disease, s.
Storm Von Leeuwen chamber
stosstherapy
Stoxil
straight (heterosexual)
stratified thrombus

streak gonads
streak plate
street
  drugs, s.
  virus, s.
strep (streptococcus)
  EIA, s.
  screen, s.
Streptase
strepticemia
streptococcal
  toxin, s.
streptococcemia
streptococcolysin
Streptococcus
  bovis, S.
  pneumoniae, S.
  pyogenes, S.
streptococcus serum
streptocolysin
streptodornase (SD)
streptohemolysin
streptokinase (SK)
  -streptodornase, s. (SKSD)
streptoleukocidin
streptolysin (SL)
  O, s.
  S, s.
streptomycin
streptosepticemia
streptozocin (STZ)
streptozotocin
stress
  polycythemia, s.
stroma
  fibrin, s.
  -free hemoglobin, s. (SFHb)
stromal cells
stromatin
stromatolysis
Strongyloides
  stercoralis, S.
strongyloidiasis
structural gene
STS (serologic test for syphilis)
STT (serial thrombin time)

Stuart factor
Stuart-Prower factor (factor X)
Stypven time test
STZ (streptozocin)
SUA (serum uric acid)
sublethal
  dose, s.
  gene, s.
subleukemic leukemia
sublocus
subpopulation
subset
substance
  abuse, s.
  P, s.
substitution transfusion
substrate
subunit vaccine
subvirion vaccine
sucrose
  hemolysis test, s.
  lysis test, s.
sucrosemia
sugar water test
sulfadiazine
sulfadoxine-pyramethamine (Fansidar)
sulfamethoxazole
sulfamethoxazole/trimethoprim
  (SMX/TMP)
sulfatemia
sulfhemoglobin
sulfhemoglobinemia
sulfinpyrazone
sulfmethemoglobin
sulfonamide
sulfonamidemia
sulpholipids
Sumatriptan
SUN (serum urea nitrogen)
supernatant
supernate
supplementary gene
suppression
suppressive therapy
suppressor
  gene, s.

146 suppressor

suppressor *(continued)*
    T-cells, s.
suppurative fever
suprapharmacologic
suramin sodium
surface
    antigen, s.
    marker, s.
Surgical Nu-Knit
Surgicel
surveillance
susceptibility
susceptible
SV (simian virus)
    40, S.
Svedberg's unit
Swan-Ganz catheter
Sweet's syndrome
swish and swallow mouthwash
Swiss-type
    agammaglobulinemia, S.
    hypogammaglobulinemia, S.
symplex
symptosis
synaptosomal/microsomal membrane
SynchroMed programmable pump
synclitic

synclitism
syncytial
syncytiolysin
syncytium
syncytoid
syndesmophyte
syndrome of sea-blue histiocyte
synergism
synergist
synergistic
synergy
syngeneic
Synkayvite
syntenic gene
synthesis
synthesize
synthetase
synthetic antigen
syntropic
syphilis
syphilitic
System 22 Mizer nebulizer
systemic
    chemotherapy, s.
    lupus erythematosus, s. (SLE)
Sytobex

Additional entries

T

13-cis-retinoic acid
T (tumor)
T2 RIA (thyroxine radioisotope assay)
T3 (triiodothyronine)
    resin uptake, T. (triiodothyronine resin uptake)
    RIA, T. (triiodothyronine radioimmunoassay)
T4 (thyroxine)
    RIA, T. (thyroxine radioisotope assay)
    surface marker, T.
T4+Leu3a+ cells
T4:T8 ratio
T8+Leu2a+ cells
TA (toxin-antitoxin)
TAA (transfusion-associated AIDS or tumor-associated antibodies)
TAB (typhoid, paratyphoid A, and paratyphoid B)
TAC antigen
Tacaribe virus
TAF (toxoid-antitoxin floccules)
tagging
T-agglutination
T-agglutinin
taheebo tea
Tahyna virus
Takayasu's arteritis
TAL (thymic alymphoplasia)
T-ALL (T-cell acute lymphoblastic leukemia)
Tamiami virus
Tamm-Horsfall mucoprotein
tandem series
tanned red cell (TRC)
    hemagglutination inhibition test, t.
T-antigen (tumor antigen—T1, T3, T4, T5, T6, T8, T9, T10, T11, T12)
TARA (tumor-associated rejection antigen)
target
    cell, t.
    erythrocyte, t.

target *(continued)*
    organ, t.
    site, t
TAR syndrome
tartaric acid solution
tart cell
TAR (thrombocytopenia-absent radius)
TASA (tumor-associated surface antigen)
TAT (toxin-antitoxin or transacting transcriptional regulation or thromboplastin activation test)
tat (transactivator)
    -3 gene, t.
TA-AIDS (transfusion-associated AIDS)
TB (tuberculosis)
    smear, T.
TBG (thyroxine-binding globulin)
TBGP (total blood granulocyte pool)
TBH (total body hematocrit)
TBI (thyroxine-binding index)
TBII (TSH-binding inhibitory immunoglobulins)
TBP (thyroxine-binding protein)
TCCL (T-cell chronic lymphocytic leukemia)
T-cell (thymus cell)
    acute lymhoblastic leukemia, T. (T-ALL)
    chronic lymphocytic leukemia, T. (TCCL)
    cytotoxicity and suppression, T. (T c/s)
    growth factor, T. (TCGF)
    helper cells. T.
    leukemia, T.
    lymphocytes, T.
    marker, T.
    mediated immunity, T. (TCMI)
    mitogens, T.
    ratio, T.
    replacing factor, T. (TRF)
    subset, T.
TCGF (T-cell growth factor)
TCH (total circulating hemoglobin)

TCMI (T-cell mediated immunity)
tcRNA (translation control RNA)
T c/s (T-cell cytotoxicity and suppression)
TCT (thrombin-clotting time)
T-cytotoxic cell
TD (tetanus-diphtheria)
TDA (TSH-displacing antibody)
T-dependent area
Tdth cells
TEA (thromboendarterectomy)
tear-shaped cells
Teceleukin
technetium
    diphosphonate, t.
    pertechnate, t.
Technetope II
Teichmann's crystals
telangiectasia
telangiectasis
telangiectatic
temperate virus
template
    bleeding time, t.
    theory, t.
TEN (toxic epidermal necrolysis)
terminal
    leukocytosis, t.
    status, t.
    transferase, t.
terminator
Teschen virus
testicular feminization
testosterone
TestPackChlamydia
tet (tetanus)
tetanic
tetanoid
tetanolysin
tetanometer
tetanus
    antitoxin, t.
    bacillus, t.
    -diphtheria, t. (TD)
    immune globulin, t.
    toxin, t.
    toxoid, t.

tetracycline
    -resistant Neisseria gonorrhoea, t.
        (TRNG)
tetrahydrocannabinol (THC)
TF (transfer factor)
TFS (testicular feminization syndrome)
TFT (trifluorothymidine)
6TG (6-thioguanine)
TGT (thromboplastin generation test OR
    time)
Thai hemorrhagic fever
thalassanemia
thalassemia
    hemoglobin C t.
    hemoglobin E t.
    hemoglobin S t.
    heterozygous t.
    homozygous t.
    intermedia, t.
    major, t.
    minor, t.
    mixed t.
    sickle cell t.
Thayer-Doisy unit
Thayer-Martin culture medium
THC (tetrahydrocannabinol)
theca
thecal
thecoma
Theiler's virus
T-helper cell
Theobald Smith's phenomenon
thermacogenesis
thermacogenetic
thermoagglutination test
thermoascus crustaceus
thermoexcitory
thermogenesis
thermogenetic
thermogenous
thermolabile hemoglobin
thermotherapy
theta antigen
thiamine
thianamycin
thiemia

thin-layer chromatography
    screen, t.
6-thioguanine (6TG)
thiokinase
thiol
thiolester
thiotepa
thiouracil
13-cis-retinoic acid
tholase
Thoma-Zeiss counting chamber
Thorn test
three-day fever
threshold
thrombasthenia
thrombectomy
thrombi (pl. of thrombus)
thrombin
    clotting time, t. (TCT)
    time, t. (TT)
Thrombinar
thrombin
    -soaked Gelfoam, t.
thrombinogen
thromboagglutinin
thromboangiitis
thrombocytapheresis
thrombocyte
thrombocythemia
thrombocytic
    leukemia, t.
    series, t.
thrombocytin
thrombocytocrit
thrombocytolysis
thrombocytopathia
thrombocytopathy
thrombocytopenia
    -absent radius, t. (TAR)
    purpura, t.
thrombocytopoiesis
thrombocytopoietic
thrombocytosis
thromboelastogram
thromboelastograph
thromboelastography

thromboembolism
thromboendarterectomy (TEA)
thrombogenesis
thrombogenic
thromboid
thrombokinase
thrombokinesis
thrombokinetics
thrombolymphangitis
Thrombolysin
thrombolysis
thrombolytic
thrombon
thrombopathia
thrombopathy
thrombopenia
thrombopenic anemia
thrombophilia
thrombophlebitis
thromboplastic
thromboplastid
thromboplastin
    activation test, t. (TAT)
    antecedent deficiency, t.
    generation test, t. (TGT)
    generation time, t. (TGT)
thromboplastinogen
thrombopoiesis
thrombopoietic
thrombopoietin
thrombosed
thrombosinusitis
thrombosis
thrombostasis
Thrombostat
thrombosthenin
thrombotest
thrombotic
    thrombocytopenic purpura, t. (TTP)
thrombotonin
Thrombo-Wellco test
thromboxane
thrombus (pl. thrombi)
    agonal t.
    annular t.
    ball t.

thrombus (pl. thrombi) *(continued)*
    blood plate t.
    blood platelet t.
    calcified t.
    canalized t.
    coral t.
    currant jelly t.
    hyaline t.
    infective t.
    laminated t.
    lateral t.
    marantic t.
    marasmic t.
    mixed t.
    mural t.
    obstructive t.
    occluding t.
    occlusive t.
    old t.
    organized t.
    pale t.
    parasitic t.
    parietal t.
    phagocytic t.
    plate t.
    platelet t.
    primary t.
    progressive t.
    propagated t.
    recent t.
    red t.
    stratified t.
    traumatic t.
    white t.
thrush
Thy-1 antigen
Thy fr 5 (thymosin fraction 5)
thymectomize
thymectomy
thymic
    alymphoplasia, t. (TAL)
    differentiation antigen, t.
    epithelial cell, t.
    humoral factor, t.
    humoral hormone, t. (thymosin)
    hypoplasia, t.

thymic *(continued)*
    peptide, t.
    polypeptide, t.
    transplantation, t.
thymidine
    diphosphate, t.
    monophosphate, t.
    -5'-triphosphate, t. (TTP)
thymine dimer
thymocyte
    mitogenic factor, t. (TMF)
    precursor, t.
thymol turbidity test
Thymolan
thymoma
thymonucleic acid
thymopathic
thymopentin
thymopoietin
thymoprivous
thymosin
    alpha 1, t.
    fraction 5, t. (Thy fr 5)
thymostimulin
thymotoxic
thymotoxin
thymulin
thymus
    cell, t. (T-cell)
    -dependent, t.
    -dependent antigen, t.
    -dependent cell, t.
    -independent, t.
    -leukemia antigen, t.
    nurse cell, t.
    -replacing factor, t. (TRF)
thymusectomy
thyroactive
thyrogenous
thyroglobulin
thyroid
    -binding inhibitory immunoglobulin, t.
    radioisotope assay, t. (TyRIA)
    -stimulating hormone, t. (TSH)
    -stimulating hormone releasing factor, t. (TSH-RF)

thyroid *(continued)*
   -stimulating immunoglobulin, t. (TSI)
thyroidectomize
thyroidectomy
thyroiditis
thyroprival
thyroprivia
thyrotoxemia
thyrotoxic
thyrotoxic serum
thyrotoxicosis
thyrotoxin
thyrotropic
thyrotropin
   -releasing factor, t. (TRF)
thyroxine (T4)
   -binding globulin, t. (TBG)
   -binding index, t. (TBI)
   -binding protein, t. (TBP)
   radioisotope assay, t. (T2 RIA or T4 RIA)
TIA (transient ischemic attack)
TIBC (total iron-binding capacity)
TIBO derivative
ticarcillin-clavulanate potassium (Timentin)
tick
   -borne, t.
Tietze's syndrome
Tilden's method
Timentin (ticarcillin-clavulanate potassium)
Timunox
T-IND cells (T-inducer cells)
T-inducer cells (T-IND cells)
tine test
Tinel's sign
Tiselius' apparatus
tissue
   bank, t.
   banking, t.
   culture medium, t.
   factor, t.
   graft, t.
   hypoxia, t.
   immunity, t.

tissue *(continued)*
   macrophage, t.
   plasminogen activator, t. (t-PA)
   polypeptide antigen, t.
   -specific antigen, t.
   thromboplastin, t.
   typing, t.
titer
titration
titremetric
titremetry
TKO-type I.V. (to keep the vein open)
TL (thymus-leukemia)
   antigen, T.
TLC G-65
TLI (total lymphoid irradiation)
T-locus
T-lymphocyte
   -subset ratio, T.
T-lymphotrophic human retrovirus (HLTV)
TMF (thymocyte mitogenic factor)
TMP/SMX (trimethoprim/sulfamethoxazole)
TNF (tumor necrosis factor)
TNI (total nodal irradiation)
TNTC (too numerous to count)
toad toxins
tobacco mosaic virus
tobramycin
Togaviridae
togavirus
Toison's solution
tolerance
   interval, t.
tolerant
tolerogen
tolerogenesis
tolerogenic
tolmetin
toluidine blue stain
TOPV (trivalent oral poliovirus vaccine)
TORCH (toxoplasmosis, rubella, cytomegalovirus, herpes simplex)
Torula
   capsulatus, T.

Torula *(continued)*
   histolytica,T.
torulosis
total
   blood granulocyte pool, t. (TBGP)
   body hematocrit, t. (TBH)
   circulating hemoglobin, t. (TCH)
   complement assay, t.
   iron-binding capacity, t. (TIBC)
   lymphoid irradiation, t. (TLI)
   nodal field, t.
   nodal irradiation, t. (TNI)
   parenteral alimentation, t. (TPA)
   parenteral nutrition, t. (TPN)
   rosette-forming cell, t. (TRFC)
tourniquet
   test, t.
   time, t.
Touton giant cell
toxanemia
toxemia
   pregnancy, t. of
toxic
   epidermal necrolysis, t. (TEN)
   granulation, t.
   hemolytic anemia, t.
   leukocytosis, t.
   shock syndrome, t. (TSS)
   shock syndrome toxin 1, t. (TSST-1)
toxicide
toxicity
toxicohemia
toxigenicity
toxignomic
toxin
   amanita t.
   animal t.
   anthrax T.
   bacterial t.
   botulinus t.
   cholera t.
   clostridial t.
   dermatonecrotic t.
   diagnostic diphtheria t.
   Dick t.
   diphtheria t.

toxin *(continued)*
   diphtheria t. for Schick test
   dysentery t.
   erythrogenic t.
   extracellular t.
   fatigue t.
   fugu t.
   fusarial t.
   gas gangrene t.
   inactivated diagnostic diphtheria t.
   intracellular t.
   plague t.
   plant t.
   pseudomonal t.
   Siga t.
   soluble t.
   staphylococcal t.
   streptococcal t.
   tetanus t.
   whooping cough
toxin-antitoxin (TAT)
toxinemia
toxinicide
toxinology
toxinosis
Toxocara
toxogen
toxogenin
toxoglobulin
toxoid
   -antitoxin floccules, t. (TAF)
   -antitoxoid, t.
toxolecithin
toxonosis
toxophil
toxophilic
Toxoplasma
   gondii, T.
toxoplasmic encephalitis
toxoplasmin
toxoplasmosis
toxoprotein
toxuria
t-PA (tissue plasminogen activator)
   inactivator, t.
TPA (total parenteral alimentation)

TPCF (Treponema pallidum complement-fixation)
TP-5
TPHA (Treponema pallidum hemagglutination assay)
TPI (Treponema pallidum immobilization)
TPIA (Treponema pallidum immobilization adherence)
T-piece (transport piece)
TPN (total parenteral nutrition)
TPT (typhoid-paratyphoid)
TR (tuberculin R)
tracer
Tracer Blood Glucose Micro-monitor
TRAIDS (transfusion-related AIDS)
tranexamic acid
transacting transcriptional regulation (TAT)
transactivate
transaminase
transcobalamin I, II
transcortin
transcript
transcriptase
    reverse test, t.
transcription
transcytosis
transduction
transfection
transfectoma
transfer
    factor, t.
    -RNA, t. (tRNA)
transferase
transferred antigen-transferred antibody reaction
transferrin
    receptor, r.
transformation
transforming gene
transfusion
    autologous t.
    cadaver blood t.
    direct t.
    exchange t.

transfusion *(continued)*
    exsanguination t.
    fetomaternal t.
    immediate t.
    indirect t.
    intraperitoneal t.
    intrauterine t.
    leukocyte t.
    massive t.
    mediate t.
    placental t.
    platelet t.
    replacement t.
    single-unit t.
    substitution t.
    whole blood t.
transfusion-associated AIDS (TAA or TA-AIDS)
transfusion reaction
    acute hemolytic t.
    allergic t.
    anaphylactic t.
    bacterial t.
    delayed hemolytic t.
    febrile nonhemolytic t.
    hemolytic t.
transfusion-related AIDS (TRAIDS)
transgenic organism
transglutaminase
Transgrow
transient
    ischemic attack, t. (TIA)
    spike, t.
transit time
transitional leukocyte
translation
    control RNA, t. (tcRNA)
translocation
transmigration
transmissible
transmission
    electron microscopy, t.
transplantation
    antigen, t.
    rejection, t.
transport

transport *(continued)*
   piece, t. (T-piece)
transposon
transsexual
   surgery, t.
transsexualism
transudate
transudation
transudative
transvector
transverse myelitis
transvestic
   fetishism, t.
transvestism
transvestite
traumatic
   arthritis, t.
   cardiac hemolytic anemia, t.
   herpes, t.
   proctitis, t.
   thrombus, t.
traumatized tissue
Travenol infuser
TRC (tanned red cell)
   antibody titer, T.
treatment IND (treatment with investigational new drugs)
Trecator SC
Treponema pallidum
   complement-fixation, T. (TPCF)
   hemagglutination assay, T. (TPHA)
   immobilization, T. (TPI)
   immobilization adherence, T. (TPIA)
treponemal
TRF (T-cell replacing factor OR thymus-replacing factor)
TRFC (total rosette-forming cell)
trialism
trialistic theory
Triboulet's test
tricholeukocyte
Trichomonas
trichomoniasis
Trichophyton
Trichosanthes kirilowii
trichosanthin

trifluorothymidine (TFT)
trifluridine
triiodothyronine
   radioimmunoassay, t. (T3 RIA)
   resin uptake, t. (T3 resin uptake)
trimellitic anhydride
trimethoprim (TMP)
   -sulfamethoxazole, t. (TMP/SX)
trimetrexate
Trimox
Trinsicon
triphthemia
triple
   antibody sandwich technique, t.
   blind, t.
   -lumen catheter, t.
   vaccine, t.
trisodium phosphonoformate (Foscarnet)
trisulfapyrimidine
tritiated thymidine
tritiation
Triton X
trivalent oral poliovirus vaccine (TOPV)
tRNA (transfer RNA)
   suppressor, t.
TRNG (tetracycline-resistant Neisseria gonorrhoea)
Trobicin
troches
trolley-track sign
trophozoite
tropical
   anemia, t.
   eosinophilia, t.
   macrocytic anemia, t.
   splenomegaly syndrome, t.
   sprue, t.
tropism
tropocollagen
Trousseau-Lallemand bodies
TruCut needle
true intersex
Trypanosoma
trypanosomiasis
trypsin
tryptase

TSA (tumor-specific antigen)
TSH (thyroid-stimulating hormone)
   -binding inhibitory immunoglobulins, T. (TBII)
   -displacing antibody, T. (TDA)
   RF, T. (thyroid-stimulating releasing factor)
TSI (thyroid-stimulating immunoglobulin)
TSS (toxic shock syndrome)
TSST-1 (toxic shock syndrome toxin 1)
TSTA (tumor-specific transplantation antigen)
T-suppressor cells
TT (thrombin time)
TTP (thymidine-5'triphosphate)
T-tube (tracheostomy tube)
TU (tuberculin unit)
tuberculin
   R, t. (TR)
   reaction, t.
   test, t.
   tine test, t.
   unit, t. (TU)
   volutin, t.
   zymoplastiche, t. (TZ)
tuberculization
tuberculocidin
tuberculoid
tuberculoidin
tuberculosis (TB)
tuberculostatic
tuberculostearic acid
tuberculotic
tuberculous
   arthritis, t.
tubulin

tuftsin
tumor (T)
   -associated antibodies, t. (TAA)
   -associated rejection antigen, t. (TARA)
   -associated surface antigen, t. (TASA)
   lysis syndrome, t.
   marker, t.
   necrosis factor, t. (TNF)
   -specific, t.
   -specific antigen, t. (TSA)
   -specific transplantation antigen, t.(TSTA)
   virus, t.
turacoporphyrin
Turk's
   cell, T.
   irritation leukocyte, T.
turnover
two-dimensional immunoelectrophoresis
Twort-d'Herelle phenomenon
two-tailed Fisher's exact test
tyloxapol
type and crossmatch
type and hold
Type C RNA tumor virus
type species
typhoid
   agglutination, t.
   fever, t.
typhus
typing
TyRIA (thyroid radioisotope assay)
tyrosine
   aminotransferase deficiency, t.
tyrosinemia
TZ (tuberculin zymoplastiche)

Additional entries

U

UA001
UBI (ultraviolet blood irradiation)
ubiquitin
U-cell lymphoma
UCHL-1 (T-cell marker)
UDP (uridine diphosphate)
UDPgalactose 4-epimerase
UDPglucose 4-epimerase
Uendex
Uganda S virus
UIBC (unsaturated iron-binding capacity)
UK (urokinase)
UK-49,858
ulitis
ultrafiltration
ultrasonic nebulizer
ultrasonography
ultrasound
Ultra-TechneKow
ultraviolet blood irradiation (UBI)
umbrella filter
UMP (uridine monophosphate)
uncomplemented
undifferentiated
   cell leukemia, u.
Undritz anomaly
unfixed human salivary gland immunofluorescence test
unheated serum reagin (USR)
unidentified reading frame (URF)
Unilab Surgibone
unilateral hermaphroditism
un-ionized hemoglobin
U937/HIV-1 cell line
unit
unitarian theory
univalent
universal
   donor, u.
   recipient, u.
unsaturated iron-binding capacity (UIBC)
unsex
unsexed
unstable hemoglobin
Uppsala virus
uratemia
urea
   frost, u.
   nitrogen, u.
Ureaplasma urealyticum
uremia
uremic
uremigenic
URF (unidentified reading frame)
uric acid
uricacidemia
uricemia
uridine
   diphosphate, u. (UDP)
   monophosphate, u. (UMP)
urinalysis
urine electrophoresis
urinemia
urobilinemia
urobilinogen
urobilinogenemia
urohematoporphyrin
urokinase (UK)
urolagnia
uroporphyrin
uroporphyrinogen
   decarboxylase, u.
   III synthase, u.
UR-2 sarcoma virus
urtica
urticant
urticaria
   pigmentosa, u.
urticarial
urticariogenic
Uruma virus
USR (unheated serum reagin)

Additional entries

V

vaccigenous
vaccinable
vaccinal
vaccinate
vaccination
vaccinator
vaccinatum
vaccine
    anaplasmosis v.
    anthrax v.
    anthrax spore v.
    aqueous v.
    attenuated v.
    autogenous v.
    bacterial v.
    bacille-Calmette-Guerin (BCG) v.
    BCG (bacille-Calmette-Guerin) v.
    bronchitis v.
    Calmette's v.
    cholera v.
    Cox v.
    diphtheria-tetanus (DT) v.
    diphtheria-tetanus-pertussis (DTP) v.
    DT (diphtheria-tetanus) v.
    DTP (diphtheria-tetanus-pertussis) v.
    duck embryo v.
    epidemic typhus fever v.
    Haemophilus B conjugate v.
    hepatitis B v.
    hepatitis B v. recombinant
    heterologous v.
    heterotypic v.
    human diploid cell rabies v. (HDCV)
    humanized v.
    influenza virus v.
    killed v.
    live v.
    measles virus v.
    meningococcal polysaccharide v.
    mixed v.
    mumps virus v.
    pertussis v.
    plague v.

vaccine *(continued)*
    pneumococcal polysaccharide v.
    poliomyelitis v.
    poliovirus v. inactivated (IPV)
    poliovirus v. live oral trivalent (TOPV)
    poliovirus v. live oral (OPV)
    polyvalent v.
    rabies v.
    replicative v.
    Rh immune globulin v.
    Rocky Mountain spotted fever v.
    rubella virus v. live
    Sabin v.
    Salk v.
    Semple v.
    sensitized v.
    smallpox v.
    split-virus v.
    subunit v.
    subvirion v.
    triple v.
    tuberculosis v.
    typhoid v.
    typhoid and parathypoid v.
    typhus v.
    viral hepatitis v.
    yellow fever v.
vaccinia
    gangrenosa, v.
vaccinia immune globulin (VIG)
vaccinia vaccine
vaccinia virus
vaccinial
vacciniform
vacciniola
vaccinization
vaccinogen
vaccinogenous
vaccinoid
vaccinostyle
vaccinotherapeutics
vaccinotherapy
vaccinum

vaculoative virus
vacuolar myelopathy
vacuolating virus
Vacutainer
vacuum phenomenon
valence
valency
validity
valinemia
VAMP (vincristine, actinomycin, methotrexate, prednisone) chemotherapy
van Bogaert's sclerosing leukoencephalitis
van den Bergh's test
Vancocin
vancomycin hydrochloride
Vansil
van't Hoff's rule
Vapo-Iso
Vaquez's disease
Vaquez-Osler disease
variability
variable region
variation
variceal
    bleeding, v.
    sclerotherapy, v.
varicella
    gangrenosa, v.
varicella virus
varicella zoster (VZ)
    immune globulin, v. (VZIG)
    virus, v. (VZV)
varicelliform
    eruption, v.
varicelloid
varices (pl. of varix)
variola
variolar
variolation
varioloid
variolous
varix (pl. varices)
vascular
    collapse, v.
    compromise, v.

vascular *(continued)*
    endothelial growth factor, v. (VEGF)
    hemophilia, v.
vascularity
vasoactive-spasmogenic mediator
vasofactive cells
vasoformative cells
vasopermeability
vasopressin
vasopressor
vasotocin
vasotribe
vasotripsy
VaxSyn
VCA (viral capsid antigen)
VCR (vincristine)
VD (venereal disease)
VDEL (Venereal Disease Experimental Laboratory)
VDG (venereal disease - gonorrhea)
VDRL (Venereal Disease Research Laboratories)
    antigen, V.
    test, V.
VDS (venereal disease - syphilis)
vection
vector
    -borne, v.
    insect v.
VEE (Venezuelan equine encephalomyelitis)
    virus, V.
Veetids
vegetable fibrin
VEGF (vascular endothelial growth factor)
veil cells
veiled cells
Velban
venacavogram
venereal
    disease, v. (VD)
    disease - gonorrhea, v. (VDG)
    disease - syphilis, v. (VDS)
    warts, v.
venesection

Venezuelan equine encephalitis (VEE)
venipuncture
venom
venothrombotic
venous
    access, v.
    assay, v.
    blood, v.
    hematocrit, v.
    hyperemia, v.
    lake, v.
    thrombosis, v.
Venuglobin I
VePesid
Vercyte
verdohemin
verdohemochromogen
verdohemoglobin
verdoperoxidase
Vermox
Versene
vertical transmission
very late-appearing antigen (VLA)
very low-density lipoproteins (VLDL)
veto cells
V factor
V genes
VH (viral hepatitis)
Vi
    agglutination, V.
    agglutinin, V.
    antigen, V.
    strain, V.
VIA (virus-inactivating agent)
vibex
vibrapuncture
vibrator
vibrio (vibriones)
vibriocidal
vibrion
    septique, v.
vibriones
vibriosis
vidarabine
Videx
vif (virion infectivity factor)

VIG (vaccinia-immune globulin)
vilona
vinblastine sulfate
Vincasar
Vincent's stomatitis
vincristine sulfate
Vira-A
viral
    arthritis, v.
    budding, v.
    capsid antigen, v. (VCA)
    culture, v.
    DNA, v.
    envelope protein, v.
    hematodepressive disease, v.
    hepatitides, v.
    hepatitis, v. (VH)
    interference, v.
    neutralization, v.
    precursor, v.
    protein, v.
    replication, v.
    ribonucleic acid, v. (VRNA)
ViraPap
Virazole
Virchow
    cell, V.
viremia
virgin B cell
viricidal
viricide
viridans streptococcus
virilescence
virilism
virility
virilization
virion
    RNA, v.
virogene
virogenetic
viroids
virology
Vironostika ELISA AIDS screening test
viropexis
viroplasm
Viroptic

virose
virosis
virostatic
virucidal
virucide
virulence
virulent
virulicidal
viruliferous
viruria
virus
    Abelson's murine leukemia v.
    acute laryngotracheobronchitis v.
    adeno-associated v.
    Aleutian disease v.
    Amapari v.
    animal v.
    arbor v.
    Argentine hemorrhagic fever v.
    attenuated v.
    Australian X disease v.
    avian E26 v.
    avian erythroblastosis v.
    B v.
    bacterial v.
    Bittner v.
    Bolivian hemorrhagic fever v.
    Brunhilde v.
    Bunyamwera v.
    Bwamba v.
    C v.
    CA (croup-associated) v.
    Cache Valley v.
    California v.
    cancer-inducing v.
    Catu v.
    CCA (chimpanzee coryza agent) v.
    Chagres v.
    Chenuda v.
    chikungunya v.
    chimpanzee coryza agent (CCA) v.
    Coe v.
    Colorado tick fever v.
    Columbia SK v.
    common cold v.
    Congo-Crimean hemorrhagic fever v.

virus *(continued)*
    coryza v.
    cowpox v.
    Coxsackie v.
    Crimean hemorrhagic fever v.
    croup-associated (CA) v.
    cytomegalic inclusion disease v.
    defective v.
    dengue v.
    DNA v.
    eastern equine encephalomyelitis (EEE) v.
    EB (Epstein-Barr) v.
    Ebola v.
    ECBO (enteric cytopathogenic bovine orphan) v.
    ECDO (enteric cytopathogenic dog orphan) v.
    ECHO (enteric cytopathogenic human orphan) v.
    ECHO 28 v.
    ECMO (enteric cytopathogenic monkey orphan) v.
    ECSO (enteric cytopathogenic swine orphan) v.
    EEE (eastern equine encephalomyelitis) v.
    EMC (encephalomyocarditis) v.
    encephalomyocarditis (EMC) v.
    enteric v.
    enteric orphan v.
    entomopox v.
    epidemic keratoconjunctivitis v.
    Epstein-Barr v. (EBV)
    equine encephalomyelitis v.
    exanthematous disease v.
    filterable v.
    filtrable v.
    fixed v.
    Germistan v.
    Graffi v.
    granulosis v.
    Guama v.
    Guaroa v.
    Hantaan v.
    Hataan v.

virus *(continued)*
    helper v.
    hemadsorption, types 1 and 2
    hemagglutinating v. of Japan
    hepadnavirus
    hepatitic C v.
    hepatitis A v. (HAV)
    hepatitis B v. (HBV)
    hepatitis delta v.
    herpangina v.
    herpes v.
    herpes zoster v.
    human immunodeficiency v. (HIV)
    human T-cell leukemia/lymphoma v.
        (HTLV)
    human T-cell lymphotrophic v.
        (HTLV)
    Ilheus v.
    infectious wart v.
    influenza v.
    iridescent v.
    Japanese B encephalitis v.
    JH v.
    Junin v.
    K v.
    Kemerova v.
    Korean hemorrhagic fever v.
    Kyasanur Forest disease v.
    Langat v .
    Lansing v.
    Lassa fever v.
    latent v.
    Latino v.
    LCM v.
    lentivirus
    Leon v.
    Lepore v.
    leukovirus
    louping ill v.
    Lunyo v.
    lymphadenopathy-associated v. (LAV)
    lytic v.
    Machupo v.
    Makonde v.
    mammary tumor v.
    Marburg v.

virus *(continued)*
    masked v.
    Mayaro v.
    McKrae strain herpesvirus
    measles v.
    Mengo v.
    milker's node v.
    MM v.
    molluscum contagiosum v.
    Moloney v.
    monkeypox v.
    Mossuril v.
    mouse mammary tumor v.
    mumps v.
    murine leukemia v.
    Murray Valley encephalitis v.
    M-25 v.
    Nakiwogo v.
    neurotropic v.
    newborn pneumonitis v.
    Newcastle disease v.
    non-A, non-B hepatitis v.
    nononcogenic v.
    Norwalk v.
    Omsk hemorrhagic fever v.
    oncogenic v.
    O'nyong-nyong v.
    ornithosis v.
    Oropouche v.
    orphan v.
    papilloma v.
    pappataci fever v.
    parainfluenza v.
    Parana v.
    parapox v.
    paravaccinia v.
    parrot v.
    pharyngoconjunctival fever v.
    Pichinde v.
    picornavirus
    Piry v.
    poliomyelitis v.
    polyoma v.
    Pongola v.
    Powassan v.
    pox v.

virus *(continued)*
    pseudocowpox v.
    psittacosis v.
    Quaranfil v.
    rabies v.
    Rauscher leukemia v.
    respiratory syncytial v. (RSV)
    retrovirus
    Rift Valley fever v.
    RNA v.
    rotavirus
    Rous-associated v. (RAV)
    Rous sarcoma v. (RSV)
    RS (respiratory syncytial) v.
    Russian spring-summer encephalitis v.
    salivary gland v.
    satellite c.
    Semliki Forest v.
    Semunya v.
    Sendai v.
    Simbu v.
    simian v.
    simian v. 40 (SV40)
    Sindbis v.
    slow v.
    Spondweni v.
    street v.
    St. Louis encephalitis v.
    SV40 (simian v. 40)
    Tacaribe v.
    Tahyna v.
    Tamiami v.
    temperate v.
    Theiler's v.
    tick-borne v.
    tobacco mosaic v.
    togavirus
    tumor v.
    2060 v.
    Uganda S v.
    Uppsala v.
    Uruma v.
    vaccinia v.
    vacuolating v.
    varicella-zoster v.

virus *(continued)*
    VEE (Venezuelan equine encephalomyelitis) v.
    visnamaedi v.
    wart v.
    WEE (western equine encephalomyelitis) v.
    Wesselsbron v.
    West Nile v.
    Wyeomyia v.
    Yale SK v.
    yellow fever v.
    Zika v.
    Zimmerman v.
virus-inactivating agent (VIA)
virus interference
virus-like
    infectious agent, v. (VLIA)
    particle, v. (VLP)
virus measles
virus neutralization test
virus-neutralizing
virusemia
virustatic
viscosity
viscous
Visidex
visnamaedi virus
vitamin
    deficiency, v.
vividialysis
vividiffusion
VLA (very late appearing antigen)
VLDL (very low-density lipoproteins)
VLIA (virus-like infectious agent)
VLP (virus-like particle)
VM-26
Voges-Proskauer test
Vollmer test
volume
    coefficient, v.
    packed red cells, v. of (VPRC)
Volutrol
Von Jaksch's anemia
von Kuppfer cells
von Willebrand's

von Willebrand's *(continued)*
  antigen, v.
  disease, v.
  factor, v. (vWF)
von Zeynek and Mencki test
vpr (viral protein r)
VP-16

VPRC (volume of packed red cells)
vpu (viral protein u)
VRNA (viral ribonucleic acid)
vWF (von Willebrand factor)
VZ (varicella zoster)
VZIG (varicella-zoster immune globulin)
VZV (varicella-zoster virus)

Additional entries

W

Waaler-Rose test
Waldenstrom macroglobulinemia
Waldeyer's ring
wandering cells
Warburg apparatus
warfarin potassium
warm
    agglutination, w.
    agglutinin, w.
    antibody, w.
    hemagglutinin,
    -reactive antibody, w.
wart
    virus, w.
Warthin's cells
Warthin-Finkeldy cells
Warthin-Starry stain
WAS (Wiskott-Aldrich syndrome)
washed clot
    platelets, w.
    red cells, w. (WRC)
Wassermann
    antigen, W.
    -fast, W.
    reaction, W.
    test, W.
wasting syndrome
water
    -borne, w.
    sports, w.
Waterhouse-Friderichsen syndrome
Watson-Ehrlich reaction
WBC (white blood cell OR white blood count)
WBC/hpf (white blood cells per high-power field)
WBF (whole-blood folate)
WBH (whole-blood hematocrit)
WC (white cell)
WCC (white cell count)
WDHA syndrome (watery diarrhea, hypokalemia, achlorhydria)
WDLL (well-differentiated lymphocytic lymphoma)
WEE (western equine encephalomyelitis) virus, W.
Wegener's granulomatosis
Weichardt's antikenotoxin
Weichbrodt test
Weigart's iron hematoxylin stain
Weil-Felix test
Weingarten's syndrome
Welcker's method
Well-Cogen
Wellcovorin
well-differentiated lymphocytic lymphoma (WDLL)
Wellferon
welt
Werlhof's disease
Wesselsbron virus
West Nile virus
Westergren
    method, W.
    sedimentation rate, W.
Western
    blot test, W.
    blotting, W.
western equine encephalomyelitis (WEE)
Wetzel test
wheal
    -erythema reaction, w.-and
    -flare reaction, w.-and
    reaction time, w.
wheat germ agglutinin
Whipple's
    disease, W.
    method, W.
white
    blood cell, w. (WBC)
    blood cells per high-power field, w. (WBC/hpf)
    blood count, w. (WBC)
    cell, w. (WC)
    cell count, w. (WCC)

white *(continued)*
  graft, w.
  thrombus, w.
whitlow
whole
  blood, w.
  -blood folate, w. (WBF)
  -blood hematocrit, w. (WBH)
  -blood transfusion, w.
  body hyperthermia, w.
  body irradiation, w.
  complement assay, w.
  complement titer, w.
  lymphocyte fraction, w. (WLF)
  saliva, w.
  whole blood
whooping cough
  toxin, w.
Widal test
Widal-Felix test
Widmark's test
Wilcoxon rank sum test
wild-type gene
Williams copulating pouch operation
Williamson's blood test
Willowbrook virus
Wills factor
Wilson's disease
Winckel disease
window-period phenomenon
Winn test
Wintrobe
  hematocrit, W.
  indices, W.
  macromethod, W.
  method, W.
Wintrobe and Landsberg's method
Wishart best
Wiskott-Aldrich syndrome (WAS)
WLF (whole lymphocyte fraction)
Wobemugos
Wolman disease
wood tick
Woods-Fildes theory
works (drug paraphernalia)
WRC (washed red cells)
wrestler's herpes
Wright
  stain, W.
  technique, W.
Wroblewski method
Wucheria bancrofti
Wu-Kabat plot
Wyeomyia virus
Wymox

Additional entries

X

xanthemia
xanthine
    oxidase inhibitor, x.
xanthogranuloma
xanthoma
xanthomatosis
xanthomatous
xanthosis
    septum nasi, x. of
X chromosome
xenembole
xenenthesis
xenoantigen
xenogeneic
    antigen, x.

xenogenesis
xenogenous
xenograft
xenon 133
X factor
X-linked
    familial hypophosphatemia, X.
    gene, X.
    hyper-IgM immunodeficiency, X.
    hypogammaglobulinemia, X.
    infantile agammaglobulinemia, X.
    lymphoproliferative syndrome, X.
XM (crossmatch)
x-ray crystallography
XXY syndrome

Additional entries

Y

Yale SK virus
Yamaguchi sarcoma virus
Ya Yan Tzu
yellow fever
   vaccine, y.
   virus, y.
Yergason's sign
Yersinia

Yersinia *(continued)*
   pestis, Y.
yersiniosis
Yersin's serum
y-interferon
Y-linked gene
yoga
yohimbine

Additional entries

Z

Zahn's lines
Zaleski's test
ZDV (zidovudine)
zeatin
zeta
    potential, z.
    sedimentation rate , z. (ZSR)
    stimulation ratio, z. (ZSR)
zetacrit
Zetafuge
zidovudine (ZDV)
Ziehl-Neelsen stain
Zieve's syndrome
ZIG (zoster immune globulin)
Zika virus
Zimmerman
    elementary particles, Z.
    virus, Z.
zinc (Zn)
ZIP (zoster immune plasma)
Zn (zinc)

zone electrophoresis
zoning
zoo-agglutinin
zooprecipitin
zooprophylaxis
zootoxin
zoster
    immune globulin, z. (ZIG)
    immune plasma, z. (ZIP)
zosteriform
Zostrix
Zovirax
ZSR (zeta sedimentation rate OR zeta stimulation ratio)
Z-technique
ZVD
Zyclast
Zyderm
zygomycosis
zymosan
zymosis

Additional entries